editors:
E. C. Huskisson - G. P. Velo

Inflammatory Arthropathies

Proceedings of a European Symposium
Monte Carlo, 1-4 October 1975

Inflammatory arthropathies

Inflammatory arthropathies

Proceedings of a European Symposium
Monte Carlo, 1–4 October 1975

Organized under the auspices of The Italian League against Rheumatism

Editors
E. C. Huskisson and G. P. Velo

 1976

Excerpta Medica – Amsterdam, Oxford

© *Excerpta Medica* 1976

International Congress Series No. 401
ISBN Excerpta Medica 90 219 0329 6
ISBN Elsevier/North-Holland 0 444 15243 1

Library of Congress Cataloging in Pàblication Data
Main entry under title:
Inflammatory arthropathies.
(International congress series; no. 401)
Includes index.
1. Arthritis-Chemotherapy-Congresses. 2. Inflammation-Congresses. 3. Antiphlogistics-Congresses. 4. Indomethacin-Therapeutic use-Congresses. I. Huskisson, E. C. II. Velo, G. P. III. Italian League against Rheumatism. IV. Series.
RC933.I48 616.7'2 76-39779
sBN 0-444-15243-1

Publisher
    Excerpta Medica
    305 Keizersgracht
    Amsterdam
    P. O. Box 1126

Sole Distributors for the USA and Canada
    Elsevier/North-Holland Inc.
    52 Vanderbilt Avenue
    New York, N. Y. 10017

Printed in The Netherlands by Hooiberg, Epe

Opening Address

D. Gigante

Istituto di Reumatologia, University of Rome, Italy

On behalf of the 'Italian League against Rheumatism' I am happy to welcome whole-heartedly all the distinguished colleagues who honour with their presence this European Symposium on Inflammatory Arthropathies.

A specially hearty welcome is also extended to the numerous journalists who are indispensable in promoting awareness of our progress and the issues involved.

Monte Carlo is a splendid setting, and it is a most agreeable duty for me to deeply thank the Government of the Principality of Monaco for the many facilities offered and the kindness shown to us.

The present Symposium is along the lines of several other similar meetings, but the extremely high calibre of the speakers and the original approach to the subject matter are sure signs of success. The direct exchange of data and observations between experts from different countries is by far the best catalyst for novel ideas and original research.

We are very grateful to Merck, Sharp and Dohme, who made possible this Symposium.

I do not want to use any of the speakers' time, so without further ado I wish you a successful meeting and declare the Symposium open.

MARCH 23, 1977

Contents

IIIA.   *Past, present and future of indomethacin*

Chairman   D. P. BARCELO
Co-chairman D. GIGANTE

IIIB.   *Past, present and future of indomethacin*

Chairman   S. DE SÈZE
Co-chairman E. C. HUSKISSON

I.   *New trends in inflammation*

Chairman   G. P. Velo
Co-chairman D. A. Willoughby

General concepts of inflammation

G. P. Velo and S. E. Abdullahi

Istituto di Farmacologia, Policlinico Borgo Roma, Verona, Italy

It is not easy to give an all inclusive definition of inflammation as for most basic concepts in pathology; with a certain approximation such a definition could be 'the local reaction to injury of living tissues, especially the small blood vessels, their contents and their associated structures'. It follows from this definition that any noxa that damages living cells and tissues can lead to an inflammatory process (infections, excessive heat and cold, irradiations, e.g. with X-rays, alkalis, acids, etc.).

The first event of the process, lasting only few seconds, is a constriction of the arterioles, the muscle fibres of which respond to nervous and chemical stimuli; this constriction is followed by vasodilatation. Because of this increased volume of blood, capillaries and venules become flushed with blood.

The venules and the capillaries later become permeable to plasma proteins, leading to an accumulation of fluids in the tissues, Majno and Palade (1961) and Majno (1965) showed with the electron microscope that plasma proteins in inflamed tissue cross the wall of venules through gaps which appear among the endothelial cells. The mechanism of the gap production is unknown; it could be due to contraction of endothelial cells, which are rich in contractile microfilaments.

It has also been shown that leukocytes leave inflamed vessels by inserting pseudopodia into the junction between endothelial cells and moving through by ameboid motion and penetrating the basement membrane (Florey, 1970). This phenomenon is known as diapedesis and, because of it, inflamed tissues are rich in leukocytes, particularly polymorphs, from the beginning of the inflammatory reaction. It is worthwhile noting that the classic mediators of inflammation, e.g. histamine, serotonin and kinins, have a weak ability to accumulate leukocytes in the inflamed tissue. Bacterial products, damaged tissue and antigen/antibody complexes cause massive leukocyte migration; these factors could act either directly on leukocytes or by activating some components of complement. Among complement system C3a and C5a, peptides split off from C3 and C5, are powerful chemotactic components; C5, C6 and C7 may also be chemotactic (Di Perri and Auteri, 1974; Favilli et al., 1975).

The mode of action of chemotactic substances is not yet clear: they probably act on the contractile microfibrils and microtubules of leukocyte cytoplasm. Chemotaxis is a complex response: leukocyte mobility is directional when there are concentration differences in chemotactic factors and random in the absence of such gradients. Chemotactic substances are mostly proteins and polypeptides; nevertheless the mechanism by which leukocytes recognize the proteins which provoke migration from the others is unknown. Generally the chemotactic substances are produced by injury, tissue damage or infection. Proteolytic enzymes may render chemotactic several protein substrates: collagenase and Hageman factor produce chemotactic peptides by acting on collagen and prekallikrein respectively. Papain and tissue proteases may have a similar action on certain IgG subtypes (Wilkinson, 1974).

Recent data show that lymphocytes, like monocytes and neutrophils, may be attracted by chemotactic substances (Wilkinson et al., 1975).

Mediators

Much research has gone into attempts to determine how the body achieves such a standard response to many diverse types of injury. This led to the investigation of chemical substances (mediators), normally present in the body, whose release or activation could cause the characteristic changes of inflammation.

The first substance recognized as a mediator was 'H-substance', probably histamine (Lewis, 1927). Since then several other mediators have been discovered (Table 1). Only some of these mediators, particularly prostaglandins, will be considered in this paper.

Histamine and serotonin

Histamine is synthesized in mast cells and basophils by decarboxylation of L-histidine. It is generally accepted that histamine is the first chemical mediator

TABLE 1

Mediators of inflammation

Agent	Origin
Complement	Reticuloendothelial cells, liver
Hageman factor (activated)	
Histamine, serotonin	Basophils, mast cells, platelets
Kinins	Plasma substrate
Leukokinins	PMNs
Lymphokines	Stimulated lymphocytes
Lysosomal enzymes	PMNs, macrophages, mast cells
Plasmin	Plasma substrate (liver)
Prostaglandins	Ubiquitous intracellular precursors
Slow reacting substance of anaphylaxis (SRS-A)	Leukocytes

to be released after inflammatory stimulus and the first for which a role in the mechanism of inflammation has clearly been established (Spector and Willough-by, 1968). Its activity is transitory and expires in a short time. Its release is only the first of a sequence of events and seems to be regulated by cellular cAMP (Bourne, 1972).

The subcutaneous injection of histamine causes increased vascular permeability (Majno and Palade, 1961). The demonstration of the participation of histamine in inflammation is based on the presence of this substance in the exudate and on the inhibition of edema by antihistamine drugs or compound 48/80. Compound 48/80 and other histamine liberators, which also release serotonin, inhibit only the early stage of increased vascular permeability (30–60 minutes).

Serotonin or 5-hydroxytryptamine (5-HT) was identified in 1954 by Erspamer from enterochromaffin cells of the intestinal tract. It derives from the hydroxylation of tryptophan to 5-hydroxytryptophan which is then decarboxylated to 5-HT. Platelets of most mammals and mast cells of rats and mice are rich in serotonin: rat peritoneal mast cells contain from 0.2 to 6.0 μg per 10^6 cells (Austen, 1971).

Serotonin, like histamine, induces an increase of vascular permeability (Majno and Palade, 1961). Injection of serotonin causes edema in rats; this effect can be antagonized by dibenamide hydrochloride and lysergic acid derivatives.

Di Rosa et al. (1971) found that in carrageenan edema the early stages depend on the simultaneous release of histamine and serotonin; in fact treatment with histamine and serotonin antagonists causes suppression of the early phase of this edema. Similar suppression of the edema occurs after depletion of histamine and serotonin prior to the injection of carrageenan.

Kinins

In 1949 Rocha e Silva et al. found that trypsin and snake venom caused the formation from blood serum of a smooth muscle-contracting substance: it was recognized as a nonapeptide called bradykinin. Bradykinin, kallidin and methionyl-lysyl-bradykinin, which are present in the blood of mammals, are formed in plasma by various enzymes, by contact with glass or charged surfaces.

Kinins have different actions, such as slow contraction of isolated ileum, increase of vascular permeability, dilatation of arterioles, hypotension and pain after injection.

Bradykinin is formed by the action of kallikrein on the precursor, kininogen. Kallikrein is present in plasma as prekallikrein which can be activated by tissue proteases, increased fibrinolytic activity, Hageman factor, and PF/dil (permeability factor) (Arrigoni Martelli, 1973). Kinins are rapidly destroyed in plasma and in other body fluids by kininases and eso-endopeptidases (Erdös and Sloane, 1962; Yang and Erdös, 1967). Kinin-inactivating activity has been observed in blood elements (Erdös and Yang, 1970) and in alveolar macrophages (Greenbaum et al., 1969).

Animals depleted of kininogens with cellulose sulphate show a decrease of the inflammatory response after carrageenan injection into the hind paw (Di Rosa and Sorrentino, 1970). This effect is evident from approximately 1 to $2\frac{1}{2}$ hours after injection.

Kinins seem to be responsible for the phase of inflammation following that of histamine and serotonin (Di Rosa et al., 1971).

Prostaglandins

In 1930 the gynecologists Kurzrok and Lieb observed that fresh human semen caused contraction and relaxation in human myometrium.

Goldblatt (1933) and Von Euler (1936) independently found a factor in human seminal liquid which contracted the plain muscle and lowered the blood pressure in laboratory animals. Von Euler named this factor 'prostaglandin' (PG), as he believed that it was produced by the prostate gland. In 1957 Bergström and Sjövall isolated PGE_1 and $PGF_{1\alpha}$ in crystalline form and in 1962 the chemical structures were reported (Bergström et al., 1962).

PGs are 20 carbon atom unsaturated hydroxy fatty acids with a cyclopentane ring at C8–C12, whose precursors are eicosatrienoic acid (dihomo-γ-linolenic acid), eicosatetraenoic acid (arachidonic acid) and eicosapentaenoic acid. Today 14 natural PGs have been identified. They are present in many mammalian tissues and have been found, as isomers, even in a coral *(Plexaura homomalla)* off the coast of Florida.

Many tissues are able to synthesize PGs from essential fatty acids. They have many pharmacological activities (Weeks, 1972) and are regulators of cell functions through the cyclic nucleotide system. Butcher and Baird (1968) reported for the first time a change (decrease) of cAMP levels in isolated fat cells by PGE_1.

Biosynthesis of PGs in cells and tissues is stimulated by hormonal, mechanical and neurological means (Ramwell and Shaw, 1970). The synthesis and release presume activation of phospholipase A_2 with formation of arachidonic acid as a substrate of PGE_2 and $PGF_{2\alpha}$ (Anderson et al., 1971) (Fig. 1). The kind and amount of PG depend on the cell substrate.

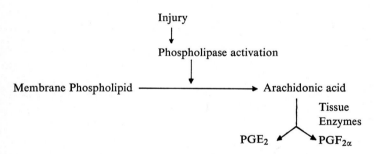

Fig. 1.   Synthesis and release of prostaglandin.

As stated above there is a relationship between PGs and the cyclic nucleotide system. PGE_1 stimulates cAMP production in human leukocytes and lymphocytes and in guinea pig granulocytes (Bourne et al., 1971; Smith et al., 1971; Stossel et al., 1970). PGE_2 is active to the same degree, while PGA_1 and $PGF_{2\alpha}$ seem to be less active; $PGF_{1\alpha}$ is almost inactive (Bourne, 1972). Like histamine, the release of PGE seems to be controlled by intracellular cAMP levels. These mediators stimulate adenyl cyclase in the cell membrane of leukocytes increasing the synthesis of cyclic AMP, which prevents a further release of histamine and PGs (Fig. 2). PGs, therefore, may act not only as mediators but also as modulators of the inflammatory reaction.

Willis (1969) has shown the presence of PGs in the late phase of foot carrageenan edema; this phase requires the presence of the complement system. Anderson et al. (1971) have found PGs (mainly PGE_2) in bleb fluid 3 hours after carrageenan, with a maximum from 12 to 24 hours; they noticed a parallel

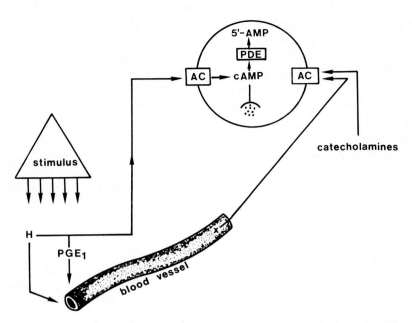

Fig. 2. Possible anti-inflammatory role of leukocyte cAMP. H = histamine; AC = adenyl cyclase; PDE = phosphodiesterase. (Modified from Bourne.)

rise of PGE_2 and β-glucuronidase. These findings have been confirmed by Velo et al. (1972).

Synovial cultures from patients suffering from rheumatoid arthritis synthesize a large amount of PGs (Robinson et al., 1973).

PGs may be inactivated quickly, after formation, by PG dehydrogenase.

Velo et al. (1973) and Willoughby et al. (1974) demonstrated that PGE_2 favours the increase of vascular permeability in carrageenan-induced pleurisy and peritonitis, whereas $PGE_{2\alpha}$ has an antagonistic effect. The antagonism between PGE and PGF_α is shown in Figure 3, which shows acute inflammation schematically. A Yin-Yang hypothesis for PGs, similar to that of Goldberg et al. (1973) for cyclic AMP and cyclic GMP (Fig. 4), could be suggested: cAMP or β-adrenergic agents, histamine and PGE_1, which accumulate cAMP, inhibit release of histamine, lymphokines, lysosomal enzymes and SRS-A; cyclic GMP or cholinergic agents and $PGF_{2\alpha}$, which accumulate cGMP, have an opposite effect. The final result would depend on the equilibrium of these two systems. Probably PGs control the release of inflammatory mediators via cyclic nucleotides which would exert their effects on the intracellular microtubules (Weissmann et al., 1971). Research on cell structure by electron

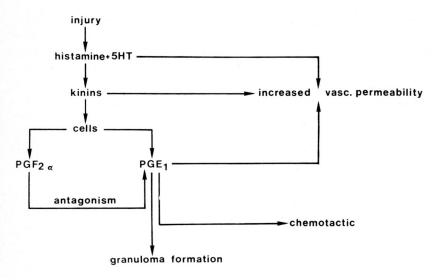

Fig. 3. Scheme of acute inflammatory process. (After Willoughby.)

microscopy suggest that PGs play a role as a controlling mechanism for ultra-structural changes in cells: they show maximal lysosomal degranulation when there is a rise of PGF relative to PGE (Velo et al., 1973).

PGs mediate the later stage of carrageenan edema (from $2\frac{1}{2}$ to 6 hours) and are associated with the migration of leukocytes into the inflamed area (Di Rosa et al., 1971). PGE_1 is chemotactic to polymorphonuclear leukocytes (Kaley and Weiner, 1971), which demonstrates a relationship between PGE and inflammatory cells. On the other hand, polymorphonuclear leukocytes release mainly PGE_2 during phagocytosis of bacteria in vitro (Higgs and Youlten, 1972).

PGs increase vascular permeability, mainly from the venules, for a longer time than histamine, and are also chemotactic to mononuclear cells (Willoughby et al., 1973). PGE_1 and $PGF_{1\alpha}$ increase collagen synthesis and enhance granuloma formation (Blumenkrantz and Søndergaard, 1972; Arora et al., 1970).

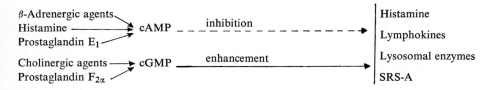

Fig. 4. Opposing actions of PGE_1 and $PGF_2\alpha$.

Because of all these characteristics, PGs seem to be implicated in the transition from acute to chronic inflammation and therefore they could perpetuate the inflammatory reaction (Velo, 1974). The inter-relationship between PGE and lymphokines would again suggest the role of the former in perpetuating inflammation. In pathological conditions, such as rheumatoid arthritis, there would be a hypersecretion of PGE and lymphokines (Morley, 1974; Bray et al., 1975).

PGE_1 and PGE_2 sensitize pain fibres and blood vessels to the effects of other mediators such as bradykinin or histamine (Ferreira and Vane, 1974).

Søndergaard and Greaves (1974) report that perfusates from the skin of patients with allergic contact eczema and primary irritant dermatitis contain PGs, which may mediate cutaneous sustained inflammation in man.

The importance of the endoperoxide system has recently become apparent (Hamberg et al., 1974). Two endoperoxides (PGG_2 and PGH_2) deriving from arachidonic acid have been studied. They have biological activities such as contraction of rabbit aorta strip and isolated guinea pig trachea, and increase of airway resistance, and induce aggregation of platelets (Samuelsson and Hamberg, 1974). PGG_2 is for the most part converted into two non-prostanoate compounds, with an oxane ring, thromboxane A_2 and thromboxane B_2, which are released in large amounts during platelet aggregation by thrombin (Samuelsson et al., 1976). This system could be implicated in the mediation and modulation of the inflammatory process.

References

ANDERSON, A. J., BROCKLEHURST, W. E. and WILLIS, A. C. (1971): Evidence for the role of lysosomes in the formation of prostaglandins during carrageenan-induced inflammation in the rat. *Pharmacol. Res. Commun.*, *3*, 13.

ARORA, S., LAHIRI, P. K. and SANJAL, R. K. (1970): The role of prostaglandin E_1 in inflammatory process in the rat. *Int. Arch. Allergy appl. Immunol.*, *39*, 186.

ARRIGONI MARTELLI, E. (1973): Biosintesi della bradichinina. In: *Aspetti di Farmacologia dell'Infiammazione*, p. 34. Tamburini Editore, Milan.

AUSTEN, K. F. (1971): Histamine and other mediators of allergic reactions. In: *Immunological Diseases*, 2nd ed., p. 332. Editor: M. Samter. Little Brown, Boston.

BERGSTRÖM, S., RYHAGE, R., SAMUELSSON, B. and SJÖVALL, J. (1962): The structure of prostaglandin E_1, F_1 and F_2. *Acta chem. scand.*, *16*, 501.

BERGSTRÖM, S. and SJÖVALL, J. (1957): The isolation of prostaglandin. *Acta chem scand.*, *11*, 1086.

BLUMENKRANTZ, N. and SØNDERGAARD, J. (1972): Effect of prostaglandins E_1 and $F_{1\alpha}$ on biosynthesis of collagen. *Nature New Biol.*, *239*, 246.

BOURNE, H. R. (1972): Leukocyte cyclic AMP: Pharmacological regulation and possible physiological implications. In: *Prostaglandins in Cellular Biology*, p. 111. Editors: P. W. Ramwell and B. B. Pharris. Plenum Press, New York–London.

BOURNE, H. R., LEHRER, R. I., CLINE, M. J. and MELMON, K. L. (1971): Cyclic 3',5'-adenosine monophosphate in the human leucocyte: synthesis, degradation and effects on neutrophil candidacidal activity. *J. clin. Invest.*, *50*, 920.

BRAY, M. A., GORDON, D. and MORLEY, J. (1975): Regulation of lymphokine secretion by prostaglandins. In: *Future Trends in Inflammation*, *II*, p. 171. Editors: J. P. Giroud, D. A. Willoughby and G. P. Velo. Birkhäuser Verlag, Basel and Stuttgart.

BUTCHER, R. W. and BAIRD, C. E. (1968): Effects of prostaglandins on adenosine 3',5' monophosphate levels in fat and other tissues. *J. biol. Chem.*, *243*, 1713.

DI PERRI, T. and AUTERI, A. (1974): On the anticomplementary action of some non-steroidal anti-inflammatory drugs. In: *Future Trends in Inflammation*, *I*, p. 215. Editors: G. P. Velo, D. A. Willoughby and J. P. Giroud. Piccin Medical Books, Padua.

DI ROSA, M., GIROUD, J. P. and WILLOUGHBY, D. A. (1971): Studies of mediators of the acute inflammatory response induced in rats in different sites by carrageenan and turpentine. *J. Path. 104*, 15.

DI ROSA, M. and SORRENTINO, L. (1970): Some pharmacodynamic properties of carrageenan in the rat. *Brit. J. Pharmacol.*, *38*, 214.

ERDÖS, E. G. and SLOANE, E. M. (1962): An enzyme in human blood plasma that inactivates bradykinin and kallidins. *Biochem. Pharmacol.*, *11*, 585.

ERDÖS, E. G. and YANG, H. Y. T. (1970): In: *Handbook of Experimental Pharmacology*, *Vol. XXV*, p. 298. Editor: E. G. Erdös. Springer Verlag, Berlin.

ERSPAMER, V. (1954): Pharmacology of indolealkylamines. *Pharmacol. Rev.*, *6*, 425.

FAVILLI, G., SPECTOR, W. G. and WILLOUGHBY, D. A. (1975): Infiammazione (o flogosi). In: *Patologia Generale*, 6th ed., p. 350. Editor: G. Favilli. Casa Editrice Ambrosiana, Milan.

FERREIRA, S. H. and VANE, J. R. (1974): Inhibition of prostaglandin biosynthesis and the mechanism of action of non-steroidal anti-inflammatory agents. In: *Future Trends in Inflammation*, *I*, p. 171. Editors: G. P. Velo, D. A. Willoughby and J. P. Giroud. Piccin Medical Books, Padua.

FLOREY, H. W. (1970): Inflammation. In: *General Pathology*, 4th ed., p. 40. Editor: H. W. Florey. Lloyd-Luke Ltd., London.

GOLDBERG, N. D., HADDOX, M. K., HARTLE, D. K. and HADDEN, J. W. (1973): The biological role of cyclic 3', 5'-Guanosine monophosphate. In: *Pharmacology and the Future of Man*, *Vol. 5: Cellular Mechanisms*, p. 146. Editor: G. H. Acheson. Karger, Basle.

GOLDBLATT, M. W. (1933): A depressor substance in seminal fluid. *J. Soc. chem. Ind.*, *52*, 1056.

GREENBAUM, L. M., FREER, R., CHANG, J., SEMENTE, G. and YAMAFUJI, K. (1969): PMN-kinin and kinin metabolizing enzymes in normal and malignant leukocytes. *Brit. J. Pharmacol.*, *36*, 623.

HAMBERG, M., SVENSSON, J. and SAMUELSSON, B. (1974): Prostaglandin endoperoxides. A new concept concerning the mode of action and release of prostaglandins. *Proc. nat. Acad. Sci. (Wash.)*, *71*, 3824.

HIGGS, G. A. and YOULTEN, L. J. F. (1972): Prostaglandin production by rabbit peritoneal polymorphonuclear leucocytes *in vitro*. *Brit. J. Pharmacol.*, *44*, 330.

KALEY, G. and WEINER, R. (1971): Effect of prostaglandin E_1 on leucocyte migration. *Nature new Biol.*, *234*, 114.

KURZROK, R. and LIEB, C. C. (1930): Biochemical studies of human semen, II. The action of semen on the human uterus. *Proc. Soc. exp. Biol. (N.Y.)*, *28*, 268.

LEWIS, T. (1927): *Blood Vessels of the Human Skin and Their Responses*. Shaw, London.

MAJNO, G. (1965): Ultrastructure of the vascular membrane. In: *Handbook of Physiology*, *Vol. 3: Section 2*, p. 2293. Editor: J. Field. Williams and Wilkins, Baltimore.

MAJNO, G. and PALADE, G. E. (1961): Studies on inflammation: I. The effect of histamine and serotonin on vascular permeability: An electromicroscopy study. *J. Biophys. Biochem. Cytol.*, *11*, 571.

MORLEY, J. (1974): Prostaglandins and lymphokines in arthritis. *Prostaglandins*, *8*, 315.

RAMWELL, P. W. and SHAW, J. (1970): Biological significance of the prostaglandins. *Rec. Progr. Hormone Res.*, *26*, 37.

ROBINSON, D. R., SMITH, H. and LEVINE, L. (1973): Prostaglandin (PG) synthesis by human synovial cultures and its stimulation by colchicine. *Arthritis Rheum.*, *16*, 129.

ROCHA E SILVA, M., BERALDO, W. T. and ROSENFELD, G. (1949): Bradykinin, a hypotensive and smooth muscle stimulating principle released from plasma globulin by snake venom and by trypsin. *Amer. J. Physiol.*, *156*, 261.

SAMUELSSON, B. and HAMBERG, M. (1974): Role of endoperoxides in the biosynthesis and action of prostaglandins. In: *Prostaglandin Synthetase Inhibitors*, p. 107. Editors: H. J. Robinson and J. R. Vane. Raven Press, New York.

SAMUELSSON, B., HAMBERG, M., MALMSTEN, C. and SVENSSON, J. (1976): The role of prostaglandin endoperoxides and thromboxanes in platelet aggregation. In: *Advances in Prostaglandin and Thrombosis Research*, *Vol. II*, p. 737. Editors: B. Samuelsson and R. Paoletti, Raven Press, New York.

SMITH, J. W., STEINER, A. L., NEWBERRY JR., W. M. and PARKER, C. W. (1971): Cyclic adenosine 3′, 5′-monophosphate in human leucocytes: alterations after phytohemagglutinin stimulation. *J. clin. Invest.*, *50*, 432.

SØNDERGAARD, J. and GREAVES, M. W. (1974): Release of prostaglandins in human cutaneous sustained inflammatory reactions. In: *Future Trends in Inflammation*, *I*, p. 45. Editors: G. P. Velo, D. A. Willoughby and G. P. Giroud. Piccin Medical Books, Padua.

SPECTOR, W. G. and WILLOUGHBY, D. A. (1968): *The Pharmacology of Inflammation*. The English Universities Press Ltd, London.

STOSSEL, T. P., MURAD, F., MASON, R. J. and VAUGHAN, M. (1970): Regulation of glycogen in polymorphonuclear leukocytes. *J. biol. Chem.*, *245*, 6228.

VELO, G. P. (1974): Co-chairman's introductory remarks. In: *Future Trends in Inflammation*, *I*, p. 3. Editors: G. P. Velo, D. A. Willoughby and J. P. Giroud. Piccin Medical Books, Padua.

VELO, G. P., BERTONI, F., CAPELLI, A. and MARTINELLI, G. (1972): Lysosomes as mediators of parenchymal lesions in adjuvant-induced arthritis in rats. *J. Path.*, *106*, 201.

VELO, G. P., DUNN, C. J., GIROUD, J. P., TIMSIT, J. and WILLOUGHBY, D. A. (1973): Distribution of prostaglandins in inflammatory exudate. *J. Path.*, *111*, 149.

VON EULER, U. S. (1936): On the specific vasodilating and plain muscle stimulating substances from accessory genital glands in man and certain animals (prostaglandin and vesiglandin). *J. Physiol. (Lond.)*, *88*, 213.

WEEKS, J. R. (1972): Prostaglandins. *Ann. Rev. Pharmacol.*, *12*, 317.

WEISSMANN, G., DUKOR, P. and ZURIER, R. B. (1971): Effect of cyclic AMP on release of lysosomal enzymes from phagocytes. *Nature new Biol.*, *231*, 131.

WILKINSON, P. C. (1974): Recognition in leucocyte chemotaxis: some observations on the nature of chemotactic proteins. In: *Future Trends in Inflammation*, *I*, p. 125. Editors: G. P. Velo, D. A. Willoughby and J. P. Giroud. Piccin Medical Books, Padua.

WILKINSON, P. C., RUSSELL, R. J., PUMPHREY, R. S. H., SLESS, F. and DELPHINE PARROTT, M. V. (1975): Studies of chemotaxis of lymphocytes. In: *Future Trends in Inflammation*, *II*. Editors: J. P. Giroud, D. A. Willoughby and G. P. Velo. Birkhäuser Verlag, Basel and Stuttgart.

WILLIS, A. L. (1969): Parallel assay of prostaglandin-like activity in rat inflammatory exudate by means of cascade superfusion. *J. Pharm. Pharmacol.*, *21*, 126.

WILLOUGHBY, D. A., GIROUD, J. P., DI ROSA, M. and VELO, G. P. (1973): The control of the inflammatory response with special reference to the prostaglandins. In: *Prostaglandins and Cyclic AMP: Biological Actions and Clinical Applications*, p. 187. Editors: R. H. Kahn and W. E. M. Lands. Academic Press Inc., New York and London.

WILLOUGHBY, D. A., GIROUD, J. P. and VELO, G. P. (1974): Progrès dans l'inflammation applicable a la polyarthrite chronique evolutive. *Bruxelles med.*, *54/3*, 135.

YANG, H. Y. T. and ERDÖS, E. G. (1967): Second kininase in human blood plasma. *Nature (Lond.)*, *215*, 1402.

Experimental acute inflammation

P. A. Dieppe

Department of Rheumatology and Experimental Pathology, St. Bartholomew's Hospital, London, United Kingdom

The acute inflammatory response is a common phenomenon, experienced by the physician in a wide variety of clinical situations. It is therefore not surprising that a large number of experimental models of the reaction have been developed. Early experiments were based on the use of a variety of nonspecific agents including thermal, chemical and physical stimuli, applied superficially to experimental animals. It was on the strength of these models that many of the basic common events in all inflammatory responses, such as the increase in vascular permeability and cellular exudation, were discovered.

Carrageenan, an extract of seaweed, was introduced as an inflammatory stimulus in 1962 (Winter et al., 1962); its introduction coincided with the appearance of indomethacin, and it was used in early work on the anti-inflammatory properties of this drug (Winter et al., 1963). Since then it has been extensively used, not only as a testing ground for new anti-inflammatory drugs, but also to investigate the mediators and cellular events in acute inflammation. Advances have come with the use of better sites for the induction of the inflammatory response as well as different agents. The use of the pleural space (Spector, 1956) allows for easy harvesting of exudate and cells for investigation. Work on carrageenan-induced foot oedema and pleurisy reactions led to current concepts of the sequence of release of the mediators of increased vascular permeability, with histamine and 5-hydroxytryptamine release being followed by a kinin phase, followed by a prolonged prostaglandin-induced phase (Di Rosa et al., 1971).

However, it has now become apparent that there are a number of problems with carrageenan. The response it produces varies from laboratory to laboratory, and is more complex than was first thought, having both complement dependent and complement independent aspects (Capasso et al., 1975). In addition we do not see people with carrageenan-induced inflammation in out-patients.

It is with this in mind that attention has turned in this laboratory to the use of inflammatory agents, and experimental models with more relevance to human diseases. Uric acid crystals, associated with gout, and calcium pyrophosphate crystals, responsible for the inflammation of 'pseudogout', have been used to produce new experimental models. The experiments to be described suggest that the nature of the agent alters the inflammatory response, so perhaps the days of the use of nonspecific models should be numbered. The clinician and the inflammologist should combine to produce models in which both the 'seed' and the 'soil' of the inflammatory reaction are as relevant as possible.

Methods

Crystals used (the 'seed'): Needle-shaped crystals of uric acid were prepared by the method of McCarty and Faires (1963). Monoclinic and triclinic crystals of calcium pyrophosphate were prepared according to the method of Brown et al. (1963). All crystals were washed 4 times, dried, and heated to 200°C for 3 hours to remove pyrogen, prior to use. The size and properties of the crystals were checked by polarising microscopy.

Sites of inflammation (the 'soil'): Five mg of crystals, suspended in 0.2 ml saline. were injected intradermally in the skin of the forearm of human volunteers. The diameter of erythema and depth of induration were measured at intervals thereafter up to 72 hours. Ten mg of crystals, suspended in 1 ml of saline, were injected into the pleural space of inbred male Wistar rats (200–250 g weight). The exudate and cells produced were harvested at intervals up to 72 hours.

Anti-inflammatory drugs: The response to indomethacin of the skin responses was assessed in 12 volunteers. Each reaction was produced twice in each person, once during a 72-hour treatment period with indomethacin, 75 mg at night and 25 mg t.d.s., and once with identical placebo treatment. The order of treatment was allocated on a random basis and the trial carried out under 'double-blind' conditions. Pleural reactions have been assessed with and without a 1-hour pre-injection dose of either indomethacin (3 mg/kg), sodium salicylate (50 mg/kg) or dexamethasone (2 mg/kg).

Results and discussion

Crystals injected intradermally in human volunteers produce an immediate area of erythema, which fades after about 1 hour; this is probably due to early release of histamine as described in the carrageenan reaction. A more prolonged phase of erythema, induration and hyperalgesia, probably related to prostaglandin release, appears some hours later. The response to uric acid is maximal at 24 hours, and that to pyrophosphate, although less marked is more prolonged, being maximal at about 36 hours. The effect of treatment with indomethacin is shown in Table 1. The diameter of erythema was significantly reduced in

TABLE 1

Response of skin reactions to indomethacin 150 mg/day in 12 male volunteers, mean of 12 observations

	Erythema		Induration	
	24 hr	48 hr	24 hr	48 hr
Uric acid				
Placebo	34.4	10.8	38.4	26.2
Indomethacin	22.5*	9.1*	33.3*	22.5
Pyrophosphate				
Placebo	13.7	5.9	11.3	7.6
Indomethacin	11.1*	4.0	11.0	7.9

*Denotes significant difference in treatment and placebo results, $p < 0.05$ (Student's 't' test).

both cases, but induration was less affected, and did not respond at all in the case of the pyrophosphate reaction. These simple experiments showed that each of the crystals produced a response with different kinetics, and suggest that their response to anti-inflammatory drugs might also vary. Further work of this sort is being carried out, and it is envisaged that models of this sort may help to develop more rational therapy for conditions like pyrophosphate arthropathy.

However, in order to investigate the mechanism of inflammation further, it is necessary to return to the animal model. Crystals injected into the pleural space of the rat induce a response maximal at 18 to 24 hours, and dominated by polymorphonuclear cells, that is, the reaction has the features of an acute inflammatory response. As in the human model urate has been found to be more active than pyrophosphate crystals of the same size and weight. Further demonstration that the model is analogous to human crystal-induced disease

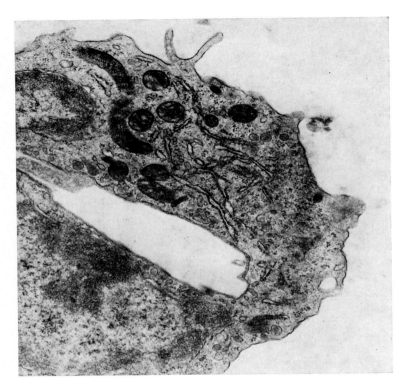

Fig. 1. A polymorphonuclear cell from a uric acid crystal induced pleural reaction, showing ingestion of a needle shaped crystal ($\times$ 21,440).

has come from study of crystal phagocytosis in the pleural model; many of the cells in the exudate contain intracellular crystals. Figures 1 and 2 show electron micrographs of polymorphonuclear cells containing uric acid and pyrophosphate crystals respectively. These appearances are similar to those described previously in gouty patients (Riddle et al., 1966; Schumacher and Phelps, 1971).

Experiments have been carried out to assess the effect of an alteration in the size and nature of the crystals on the pleural reaction. The effect of different sizes of uric acid crystal are shown in Figure 3. Powder produces a negligible reaction; crystals with an average length of 20 microns produce some effect, but a much greater response is observed with crystals of about 5 microns in length, the size of crystals found in the synovial fluid of gouty patients. This probably reflects the ability of the cells to phagocytose only those crystals of the smaller size range. In the case of pyrophosphate, a comparison has been made between a preparation predominating in monoclinic crystals and one

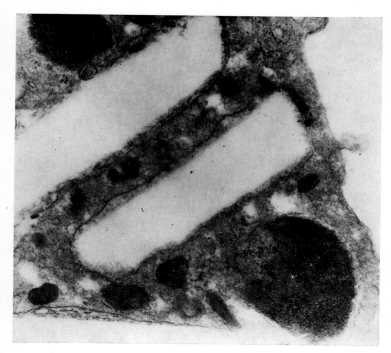

Fig. 2. Part of a polymorphonuclear cell from a pyrophosphate-induced pleural reaction, showing a membrane surrounding an ingested monoclinic calcium pyrophosphate crystal (× 33,500).

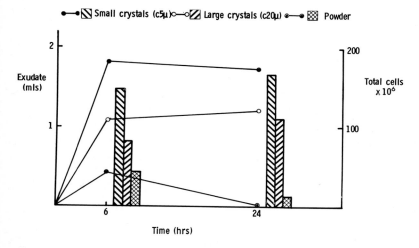

Fig. 3. The intrapleural inflammatory response to uric acid crystals of varying size.

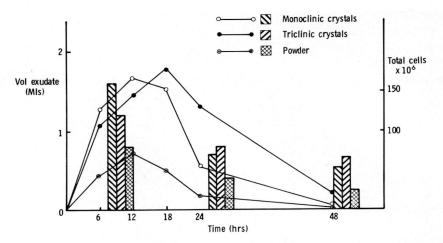

Fig. 4. The intrapleural inflammatory response to different forms of calcium pyrophosphate.

predominating in the triclinic form. As shown in Figure 4, the former produced a more acute reaction than the latter, and both were more active than powder. These results indicate that the kinetics of the inflammatory response are very dependent on the exact nature of the stimulus.

The effect of the nature of the irritant on the amount of suppression of the responses by anti-inflammatory drugs is also being assessed. Uric acid crystals coated with pyrogen have been found to produce a reaction unresponsive to either salicylate or indomethacin, whereas pyrogen-free crystal reactions are sensitive to both these drugs. Current experiments with pyrophosphate are even more interesting. In one experiment, 2 preparations, both of them lacking in complete purity, were compared. The reactions produced were both inhibited by dexamethasone, but whereas one only responded to salicylate and not to indomethacin, the other only responded to the indomethacin. These results are only preliminary, but they again emphasise the need for careful standardisation of the inflammatory stimulus if meaningful results are to be obtained. They also call into question single theories to explain the action of all anti-inflammatory drugs, such as the current theories concerning prostaglandin synthetase.

Conclusions

Research into the acute inflammatory reaction has reached a point where generalisations should no longer be made. It is clear from the above experiments that the reactions are very dependent on the exact nature of the irritant used. In view of this the inflammologist should be working with the clinician to produce models of inflammation that have direct relevance to human disease. Where possible, both the 'seed' and the 'soil' of the reaction should have an analogy in human pathology. The mechanism and the pharmacology of these models should be discussed in the setting of a particular disease. Only then will useful knowledge concerning the various inflammatory diseases and their therapy be advanced.

Acknowledgments

I wish to acknowledge the support of the Joint Research Board of St. Bartholomew's Hospital. I would like to thank Mrs C. Stevens for technical help and Mr P. Crocker and Miss G. Tyler for help with the electron micrographs and illustrations. Acknowledgment is also given to the Occupational Health Service of the Post Office, and volunteers from the East Central District Office and Foreign Section, King Edward Building, London E.C.1. for their cooperation.

References

BROWN, E. H., LEHR, J. R., SMITH, J. P. and FRAZIER, A. W. (1963): The preparation and characterisation of some calcium pyrophosphates. *J. Agric. Food Chem.*, *11*, 215.

CAPASSO, F., DUNN, C. J., YAMAMOTO, S., WILLOUGHBY, D. A. and GIROUD, J. P. (1975): Further studies on carrageenan induced pleurisy in rats. *J. Path.*, *116*, 117.

DI ROSA, M., GIROUD, J. P. and WILLOUGHBY, D. A. (1971): Studies of the mediators of the. acute inflammatory response induced in different sites by carrageenan and turpentine. *J. Path.*, *104*, 15.

MCCARTY, D. J. and FAIRES, J. S. (1963): A comparison of the duration of local anti-inflammatory effects of several adrenocorticosteroid esters – a bioassay technique. *Curr. ther. Res.*, *5*, 284.

RIDDLE, J. M., BLUHM, G. B. and BARNHART, M. L. (1966): The ultrastructure of exudative leucocytes in gout and pseudogout. *Arthr. and Rheum.*, *9*, 872.

SCHUMACHER, H. R. and PHELPS, P. (1971): Sequential changes in human polymorphonuclear leukocytes after urate crystal phagocytosis. *Arthr. and Rheum.*, *14*, 513.

SPECTOR, W. G. (1956): The mediation of altered capillary permeability in acute inflammation. *J. Path.*, *72*, 367.

WINTER, C. A., RISLEY, E. A. and NUSS, G. W. (1962): Carrageenan induced oedema in the hind paw of the rat as an assay for anti-inflammatory drugs. *Proc. Soc. exp. Biol. (N.Y.)*, *111*, 544.

WINTER, C. A., RISLEY, E. A. and NUSS, G. W. (1963): Anti-inflammatory and antipyretic activities of indomethacin, 1-(p-chlorobenzyl)-5-methoxy-2-methylindole-3-acetic acid. *J. Pharmacol. exp. Ther.*, *141*, 369.

Cellular pharmacokinetics in inflammation[*]

C. J. Dunn, J. P. Giroud and D. A. Willoughby

Department of Pharmacology, ERA 629 CNRS, Faculté de Médecine, Cochin-Port Royal, Paris, France, and Department of Experimental Pathology, St. Bartholomew's Hospital Medical College, London, United Kingdom.

In most studies on pharmacological mediators in inflammation the emphasis has been placed either on the extracellular or whole tissue content of these substances. This has arisen largely because of the difficulty in separation of the various elements at the inflammatory site. To overcome this problem, several different types of inflammation have been developed in the pleural cavity of rats and guinea-pigs. They lend themselves not only to a more precise quantitation of the oedematous and cellular phases of inflammation but also to analysis of the mediators present. This communication concentrates on the intracellular mediator levels during both immunological and non-immunological inflammatory reactions.

'Arthus' pleurisy

Arthus pleural reactions were induced by intravenous injection of bovine serum albumin (BSA) followed 20 minutes later by intrapleural challenge with purified anti-BSA antibody, according to the technique of Yamamoto et al. (1975a).

[*]Financial support was given by The European Biological Research Association (EBRA), SORBA (France), INSERM (France), CNRS (France), The Wellcome Trust, the Arthritis and Rheumatism Council.

The cellular reaction is dominated by polymorphs which attain their peak response as early as 6 hours (Table 1). The formation of fluid exudate is also immediate in onset reaching maximum levels around 6 hours (Table 1). By 24 hours the reaction has diminished considerably (Table 1). This particular reaction has also been shown to be independent of the complement system as demonstrated by depletion of circulating complement levels by pretreatment with cobra venom factor, a substance which depletes C'3–C'9 (Yamamoto et al., 1975a).

TABLE 1

Development of the reverse passive Arthus reaction in the rat pleural cavity – analysis of mediator content in the cellular exudate fraction

	Exudate collected at time (hr)					
	1	3	6	12	24	48
Vol. fluid exudate (ml)	—	—	1.95	0	0	0
Total polys, $\times\ 10^6$	—	—	60	45	17	10
Total monos, $\times\ 10^6$	—	—	20	46	40	23
Histamine, $\mu g/10^8$ cells	60.0	40.0	9.0	1.0	1.0	0
5-HT, $ng/10^8$ cells	50	10	15	10	11	5
PGE_2, $ng/10^8$ cells	0	6	4.2	2.3	3.2	0
$PGF_{2\alpha}$, $ng/10^8$ cells	1	2	2.7	6.0	3.2	2.0

Delayed hypersensitivity

Another immunological model which has been successfully induced in the pleural cavity of guinea-pigs is that of delayed hypersensitivity (DH) to tuberculin. The reaction is induced by sensitising guinea-pigs with comple Freunds adjuvant followed 3 weeks later by intrapleural challenge with PPD (Yamamoto et al., 1975b). Measurement of increased vascular permeability was carried out by estimation of the leakage of I^{125}-labelled guinea-pig IgG into the pleural cavity. Table 2 shows that the onset of the formation of fluid exudate and increased vascular permeability is delayed in contrast to the Arthus reaction, the peak response being attained between 12 and 18 hours. This delayed characteristic is also reflected in the cellular reaction which reaches maximal levels between 18–24 hours (Table 3). In contrast to the Arthus reaction, that of DH is typified by a predominance of mononuclear cells among which both monocytes and lymphocytes are found (Table 3).

A further distinction between the Arthus and DH pleural reactions was that the latter was found to be unaffected by the depletion of complement and thus thought to be independent of this system (Yamamoto et al., 1975b).

TABLE 2

Quantitation of exudate induced by intrapleural injection of PPD into CFA-sensitised guinea-pigs

No. of animals	Exudate collected at time (hr)	Volume exudate (ml)	S.E.	^{125}I IgG (cell-free exudate) (c.p.m.)
10	1	0.3	($\pm$ 0.2)	—
18	6	0.7	($\pm$ 0.3)	821
18	12	2.3	($\pm$ 1.5)	3750
18	18	5.0	($\pm$ 1.9)	3190
19	24	3.5	($\pm$ 1.2)	1914
16	30	2.0	($\pm$ 0.9)	—
16	48	0.5	($\pm$ 0.6)	520

(From Yamamoto et al., 1975b.)

TABLE 3

Development of the delayed hypersensitivity reaction in the pleural cavity of the guinea-pig – analysis of mediator content in the cellular exudate fraction

	Exudate collected at time (hr)						
	1	3	6	12	18	24	48
Vol. fluid exudate (ml)	0	0.2	0.4	3.1	5.0	4.4	0.7
Total polys, $\times$ 10^6	—	—	11	20	43	48	15
Total monos, $\times$ 10^6	—	—	8	19	45	52	24
Histamine, ng/10^8 cells	60	100	160	122	—	64	56
5-HT, ng/10^8 cells	5	0	0	0	0	0	0
PGE$_2$, ng/10^8 cells	0	0	1.0	3.5	—	1.2	1.0
PGF$_{2\alpha}$, ng/10^8 cells	0	0	1.0	7.0	—	4.0	4.5

Analysis of histamine, 5-HT, PGE$_2$ and PGF$_{2\alpha}$ in various pleural exudates

The mediators histamine, 5-HT and prostaglandins E$_2$ and F$_{2\alpha}$ (PGE$_2$, PGF$_{2\alpha}$), were measured both in the cell fraction ('intracellular') and in the cell-free fraction ('extracellular') of the various inflammatory pleural exudates. Extracellular levels, although not reported here, followed essentially the same pattern as for the respective intracellular levels.

(a) Arthus pleurisy. For the Arthus pleural reaction both histamine and 5-HT reach maximum levels around 1 hour after challenge and thereafter rapidly subside (Table 1). PGE_2 levels follow a similar pattern reaching a peak around 3 hours (Table 1). Thus these 3 mediators of increased vascular permeability may be responsible for the initial exudate induced during the Arthus reaction since their maximal levels closely precede peak exudate formation (i.e. around 6 hours). However, $PGF_{2\alpha}$ rises more slowly, reaching its highest level around 12 hours (Table 1). Such an observation may explain the termination of exudate formation by $PGF_{2\alpha}$ since this prostaglandin has been found to inhibit vascular permeability induced by PGE_2 in vivo (Willoughby, 1968). In this context PGE_2 may be considered as pro-inflammatory and $PGF_{2\alpha}$ anti-inflammatory.

(b) Carrageenan pleurisy. The mediators of carrageenan pleurisy were also measured since this reaction, like that of the Arthus, is complement-dependent (Capasso et al., 1975). Both histamine and 5-HT were detected in the carrageenan-induced pleural exudates and were observed to reach peak levels around 1 hour as in the Arthus reaction (Table 4). Similarly, these observations were made prior to the development of maximum exudate formation, suggesting a role for histamine and 5-HT in the induction of increased vascular permeability by carrageenan, as previously suggested by Di Rosa et al. (1971) using the rat hind paw test of Winter et al. (1962). PGE_2, which is initially higher than $PGF_{2\alpha}$, is as pronounced as in the Arthus reaction, although its peak is found at the later time of 12 hours. Nevertheless, $PGF_{2\alpha}$ rises as the exudate wanes, further reinforcing its possible role as an inhibitor of increased vascular permeability (Table 4).

TABLE 4

Development of the carrageenan reaction in the rat pleural cavity – analysis of mediator content in the cellular exudate fraction

	Exudate collected at time (hr)					
	1	3	6	12	24	48
Vol. fluid exudate (ml)	—	—	2.0	—	0.9	0
Total polys, $\times\ 10^6$	—	—	86	—	53	30
Total monos, $\times\ 10^6$	—	—	38	—	36	32
Histamine, $\mu g/10^8$ cells	9.6	4.0	3.6	5.5	4.5	3.7
5-HT, $ng/10^8$ cells	10.2	4.3	6.0	2.5	5.4	5.4
PGE_2, $ng/10^8$ cells	1.8	2.4	5.0	7.0	5.3	5.6
$PGF_{2\alpha}$, $ng/10^8$ cells	0	1.0	6.5	8.4	12.0	11.0

(c) Delayed hypersensitivity. Neither histamine nor 5-HT were found in significant amounts at any time during the DH reaction which was in marked contrast with the complement-dependent reactions (i.e. Arthus, carrageenan) (Table 3). Thus it is unlikely that either of these 2 mediators contribute to increased vascular permeability in the DH reaction. PGE_2 appears more closely related to the development of increased vascular permeability in this reaction (Table 3). However, $PGF_{2\alpha}$, which has already been shown to inhibit PGE_2-induced vascular permeability, is found in higher concentration than PGE_2 from 6 hours onwards (Table 3). Thus, if $PGF_{2\alpha}$ possesses this activity in an inflammatory exudate it would appear unlikely that PGE_2 would be active during this time.

(d) Calcium pyrophosphate dihydrate. Comparison of the DH pleurisy with that induced by calcium pyrophosphate dihydrate (CPPD, another complement-independent reaction – see Willoughby et al., 1975) revealed essentially the same findings with respect to histamine and 5-HT (Table 5). These mediators were barely detectable during the CPPD reaction and their significance was therefore thought to be negligible. As with the different pleural reactions mentioned above, the rise in $PGF_{2\alpha}$ above that of PGE_2 occurred during the later stages of the reaction and was coincident with the decrease in exudate formation (Table 5).

Analysis of cyclic AMP in various pleural reactions

Cyclic AMP (cAMP) was assayed for both cellular ('intracellular') and cell-

TABLE 5

Development of the calcium pyrophosphate dihydrate (CPPD) reaction in the rat pleural cavity – analysis of mediator content in the cellular exudate fraction

	Exudate collected at time (hr)					
	1	3	6	12	24	48
Vol. fluid exudate (ml)	—	—	1.9	—	0.5	0
Total polys, $\times 10^6$	—	—	55	—	45	15
Total monos, $\times 10^6$	—	—	20	—	32	10
Histamine, $ng/10^8$ cells	2.5	2.0	2.0	1.9	1.1	0
5-HT, $ng/10^8$ cells	1.0	1.0	0	0	0	0
PGE_2, $ng/10^8$ cells	0	1.0	2.7	2.7	2.3	2.2
$PGF_{2\alpha}$, $ng/10^8$ cells	0	0	2.6	6.8	14.3	2.1

free ('extracellular') exudate. Extracellular cAMP levels followed the same pattern as for intracellular levels and only the latter are therefore reported here. For each type of inflammatory reaction an initial fall in cAMP was observed followed by a rise to, or above, normal levels as each reaction diminished (Table 6). Thus, no difference was observed between the 4 types of reaction studied. An inverse correlation between cAMP levels and the intensity of the inflammatory response was consistently observed, irrespective of its immunological/non-immunological nature or even its complement dependence.

TABLE 6

Quantitation of cAMP concentration in the cellular exudate fraction of various experimental pleurisies

Type of reaction	cAMP (pmoles/10^8 cells) measured at time (hr)							
	0	1	3	6	12	18	24	48
Carrageenan (rat)	180	—	65	130	—	420	670	470
CPPD (rat)	280	—	85	105	120	—	193	281
Arthus (rat)	165	133	30	50	64	—	130	360
DH (guinea-pig)	95	120	—	34	—	34	24	67

These findings are of considerable importance in view of recent observations which suggest that cAMP is anti-inflammatory. Thus, it has been shown that increased intracellular cAMP may lead to inhibition of the following processes in vitro: lymphocyte transformation (Hirschhorn et al., 1970; Smith et al., 1971) and cytotoxicity (Strom et al., 1973); mediator release during 'in vitro' anaphylaxis (Kaliner and Austen, 1974, 1975); platelet aggregation (Vigdahl et al., 1969; Bruno et al., 1974); lysosomal enzyme release from mixed human leucocyte populations (Weissmann et al., 1973; Zurier et al., 1974; Ignarro, 1974). Thus the rise in cAMP found towards the end of each pleural reaction may reflect the role of this nucleotide as an anti-inflammatory mediator in an attempt to terminate the reaction. Its function in both the Arthus and carrageenan reactions may be particularly significant with respect to inhibition of histamine release as found in the 'in vitro' anaphylactic reaction by Kaliner and Austen (1974, 1975). For the DH reaction the significance of the late rise in cAMP may well reflect an inhibition of lymphocyte transformation as observed by Hirschhorn et al. (1970) and Smith et al. (1971) 'in vitro'.

In each of the 4 types of inflammatory reaction the rise in cAMP may serve a general purpose, i.e. that of inhibition of lysosomal enzyme secretion by leucocytes as described 'in vitro' by Weissmann et al. (1973) and Zurier et al. (1974). Whatever the precise role of cAMP in inflammation the results reported here 'in vivo' tend to support those of 'in vitro' work. However, there remain several unanswered questions.

PGE is one of many substances which may stimulate increased intracellular cAMP in leucocytes (Weissmann et al., 1973; Kaliner and Austen, 1974, 1975). It has been reported in this communication that the highest PGE levels were found in the early stages of all 4 types of inflammatory reaction tested. It is therefore difficult to ascertain the exact role of PGE 'in vivo', which on the one hand is pro-inflammatory (via increased vascular permeability) and yet on the other hand should be anti-inflammatory (i.e. via increased cAMP). The latter property of PGE is certainly not evident 'in vivo'. However, there are other substances which may stimulate the formation of intracellular cAMP in leucocytes such as β-adrenergic agents (Weissmann et al., 1973; Kaliner and Austen, 1974, 1975). It would be of interest to determine the activity of these substances during the later stages of the inflammatory reaction. This possibility remains to be explored further with the use of the various models of pleural inflammation described above.

References

BRUNO, J. J., TAYLOR, L. A. and DROLLER, M. J. (1974): Effects of PGE$_2$ on human platelet adenyl cyclase en aggregation. *Nature, (Lond.)*, *251*, 721.

CAPASSO, F., DUNN, C. J., YAMAMOTO, S., WILLOUGHBY, D. A. and GIROUD, J. P. (1975): Further studies on carrageenan-induced pleurisy in rats. *J. Path.*, *116*, 117.

DI ROSA, M., GIROUD, J. P. and WILLOUGHBY, D. A. (1971): Studies of the mediators of the acute inflammatory response induced in rats in different sites by carrageenan and turpentine. *J. Path.*, *104*, 15.

HIRSCHHORN, R., GROSSMAN, J. and WEISSMANN, G. (1970): Effect of 3'5'-adenosine monophosphate and theophylline on lymphocyte transformation. *Proc. Soc. exp. Biol. (N.Y.)*, *133*, 1361.

IGNARRO, L. J. (1974): Regulation of lysosomal enzyme secretion: role in inflammation. *Agents and Actions*, *4*, 241.

KALINER, M. and AUSTEN, K. F. (1974): Cyclic AMP, ATP and reversed anaphylactic histamine release from rat mast cells. *J. Immunol.*, *112*, 664.

KALINER, M. and AUSTEN, K. F. (1975): Immunologic release of chemical mediators from human tissues. *Ann. Rev. Pharmacol.*, *15*, 177.

SMITH, J. W., STEINER, A. L. and PARKER, C. W. (1971): Human lymphocyte metabolism. Effects of cyclic and non-cyclic nucleotides on stimulation by phytohaemagglutinin. *J. clin. Invest.*, *50*, 442.

STROM, T. B., CARPENTER, C. B., GAROVOY, M. R., AUSTEN, K. F., MERRILL, J. P. and KALINER, M. (1973): The modulating influence of cyclic nucleotides upon lymphocyte-mediated cytotoxicity. *J. exp. Med.*, *138*, 381.

VIGDAHL, R. L., MARQUIS, N. R. and TAVORMINA, P. A. (1969): Platelet aggregation: adenyl cyclase PGE$_1$ and calcium. *Biochem. biophys. Res. Commun.*, *37*, 409.

WEISSMANN, G., ZURIER, R. B. and HOFFSTEIN, S. (1973): Leucocytes as secretory organs of inflammation. *Agents and Actions*, *3*, 370.

WILLOUGHBY, D. A. (1968): Effects of prostaglandins PGF$_{2\alpha}$ and PGE on vascular permeability. *J. Path.*, *96*, 381.

WILLOUGHBY, D. A., DUNN, C. J., YAMAMOTO, S., CAPASSO, F., DEPORTER, D. A. and GIROUD, J. P. (1975): Calcium pyrophosphate induced pleurisy in rats: a new model of acute inflammation. *Agents and Actions*, *5*, 35.

WINTER, C. A., RISLEY, E. A. and NUSS, G. W. (1962): Carrageenan-induced oedema in the hind paw of the rat as an assay for anti-inflammatory drugs. *Proc. Soc. exp. Biol. (N.Y.)*, *111*, 544.

YAMAMOTO, S., DUNN, C. J., DEPORTER, D. A., CAPASSO, F., WILLOUGHBY, D. A. and HUSKISSON, E. C. (1975a): A model for the quantitative study of Arthus (immunologic) hypersensitivity in rats, *Agents and Actions*, *5*, 374.

YAMAMOTO, S., DUNN, C. J., CAPASSO, F., DEPORTER, D. A. and WILLOUGHBY, D. A. (1975b): Quantitative studies on cell-mediated immunity in the pleural cavity of guinea-pigs. *J. Path.*, *117*, 65.

ZURIER, R. B., WEISSMANN, G., HOFFSTEIN, S., KAMMERMAN, S. and TAI HSIN HSIUNG (1974): Mechanisms of lysosomal enzyme release from human leukocytes. II. Effects of cyclic AMP and cyclic GMP, autonomic antagonists and agents which affect microtubule function. *J. clin. Invest.*, *53*, 297.

Inhibition of prostaglandin biosynthesis as the mechanism of action and the therapeutic effect of non-steroid anti-inflammatory agents

S. H. Ferreira

Department of Pharmacology, Faculty of Medicine of Ribeirão Preto, São Paulo, Brazil

The basic hope scientists have is that of being able to control phenomena instead of merely leaving them to run their natural course. Obviously the best way of intervening in an inflammation is to minimize the trauma responsible for the ongoing tissue injury (Fig. 1, (1)). Because salicylates suppress a variety of reactions in vivo which have an immunological basis (allergic encephalomyelitis in the guinea pig, serum sickness in man, reverse passive Arthus in rabbit, etc), much attention has been directed to their effect on antigen-antibody reactions. Although the effects of salicylates on a variety of systems is well established in vitro, there is no good evidence in vivo that support this mechanism. Another popular thought regarding the site of action of aspirin-like drugs has been a possible interference with leucocytes, such as the inhibition of their migration (Di Rosa et al., 1971a, b) or phagocytosis (Chang, 1972). However, those drugs do not affect their migration (for discussion, see Van Arman and Carlson, 1973) or the release of lysosomal enzymes expected during phagocytosis (Willis et al., 1972).

In Figure 1 we made an attempt to cluster the main possible sites of action of anti-inflammatory drugs. Among the several hypotheses advanced to explain the action of aspirin-like drugs, inhibition of oxidative phosphorylation has

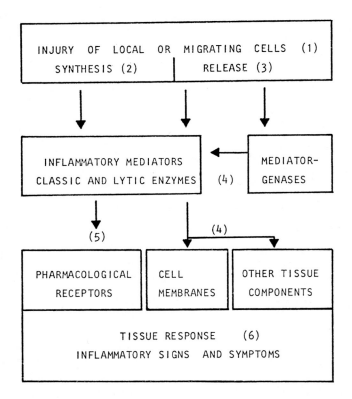

Fig. 1. Possible sites of action of anti-inflammatory drugs. A trauma may cause an injury of local or migrating cells. The trauma (1) responsible for the ongoing injury can be minimised: (a) by interfering with the formation of the effective traumatic stimulus. This is for example the case of agents which block the formation of immuno-complexes or inhibit the formation of urate crystals into the joints: (b) by protecting cells from the trauma, like the dusting powders; and (c) by reducing migrating cells, thus lowering the intensity of the inflammatory reaction, like methotrexate.

Injured cells may inhibit (a) the synthesis of substances such as prostaglandins (2); this is the case with aspirin-like drugs; (b) the release of preformed active substances, lysosomes, enzymes and pre-kallikreins. The interaction antigen-antibody is ineffective to release histamine. In the presence of Intal the release of enzymes is thought to be blocked by corticoids. Released enzymes may generate mediators (such as kallikreins) or directly damage tissue components. Thus, inhibition of enzymes block either the formation of mediators (this is the case with trasylol on the kallikrein system) or the direct action of the enzymes (nowadays there is a search for agents able to inhibit phospholipases and collagenase). Most of the inflammatory signs and symptoms are induced by the action of mediators on the cell membrane receptors. There are few mediator antagonists (5) which are effective in inflammation (antihistaminics and anti-5-hydroxytryptamine drugs). It is thought that the anti-inflammatory action of corticoids is to depress the response of the effector cells to the inflammatory mediators (6).

caused some stir, but no convincing evidence relating uncoupling potency to anti-inflammatory activity has been obtained (Smith and Dawkins, 1971). In fact it is difficult to understand how a general inhibition of oxidative phosphory-lation could modify the course of an inflammation without being detrimental to the animal. One needs to suppose that this effect is cell-specific, acting for example in the migrating cells (Fig. 1 (1)) or modifying the response of the effector cells involved in the generation of inflammatory signs and symptoms Fig. 1 (6)). This last mechanism does not seem to be valid, since aspirin does not substantially alter the oedema produced by dextran, passive cutaneous anaphylaxis or that observed during the first phase of an inflammation caused by a mixture of carrageenan and prostaglandins (see below).

Since a cardinal feature of acute inflammation is fluid exudate, secondary to increased capillary permeability, attention has been devoted to the possi-bility that aspirin-like drugs could be acting by blocking the formation (Fig. 1 (2)), release (3) or action (5) of local tissue mediators. Aspirin-like drugs do not suppress bradykinin formation or prevent the increased vascular permeability induced by it. The same can be said with regard to 5-hydroxytryptamine and histamine.

Inhibition of the biosynthesis of prostaglandin was recently proposed as the mode of action of aspirin-like drugs (Vane, 1971; Smith and Willis, 1971; Ferreira et al., 1971). After 5 years the strength of this hypothesis lies not only in the fact that non-steroid drugs inhibit the generation of prostaglandins in vitro and in vivo in a multitude of preparations but also on the growing evidence that prostaglandins play a part in the genesis of pain, fever and inflammatory oedema. This paper is a brief review of the action of the non-steroid anti-inflammatory drugs upon the prostaglandin synthetase enzymes. It also analyses the contribution of prostaglandins to the development of inflammatory signs and symptoms (for more detailed reviews, see Ferreira and Vane, 1974 a, b).

Inhibition of prostaglandin synthetase

Since it was shown that aspirin-like drugs inhibit the prostaglandin synthetases from man, dog and guinea pig, this anti-enzyme action has been amply con-firmed and demonstrated in many biological preparations and in almost all laboratory species like cat, rat, gerbil, mouse, sheep, dog, rabbit, bull and sheep. The absolute potency of the non-steroid anti-inflammatory drugs against prostaglandin synthetase varies not only with the source of the enzyme pre-paration but also with experimental conditions and the way in which the en-zyme is prepared (Flower and Cheung, 1973; Ham et al., 1972; Takeguchi and

Sih, 1972). However, in general, the overall rank order of potency is independent of the enzyme preparation, although there are some minor variations (even when the same preparation is used; Flower and Cheung, 1973). Variations in activity relative to each other will be discussed below.

Despite these variations in potency, inhibition of prostaglandin biosynthesis is clearly a general characteristic of aspirin-like drugs. It also seems to be a unique characteristic, for compounds selected to represent many other types of pharmacological activity were inactive ($< 10\%$ inhibition at 100 μg/ml). These included chloroquine, morphine, mepyramine, probenecid, azathioprine, para- and meta-hydroxybenzoic acid, Phenergan, atropine, methysergide, phenoxybenzamine, propranolol, iproniazid, droperidol, chlorpromazine and disodium cromoglicate (Vane 1971; Flower et al., 1972).

Several papers have compared anti-inflammatory activity of aspirin-like drugs with their activity against prostaglandin synthetase. A good correlation is evident, even when comparison is based on oral administration of the drug on the one hand and direct inhibition of an in vitro microsomal enzyme preparation on the other. The rank order was the same against carrageenan rat paw oedema as against the spleen synthetase, except that indomethacin was out of order for the rat paw test (Flower et al., 1972). Even more striking is the correlation shown by comparing pairs of enantiomers. This has been done for naproxen and for indomethacin analogues. In each instance, the one of each pair with anti-inflammatory activity also strongly inhibited prostaglandin synthetase, whereas the one with weak anti-inflammatory activity was also weak against the synthetase (Tomlinson et al., 1972; Ham et al., 1972).

Recently, we (Ferreira et al., 1975a) described a method in which inflammatory exudates were induced in rats by subcutaneous implantation of sponges impregnated with carrageenan. It was possible to correlate inhibition in vivo of prostaglandin synthesis and anti-inflammatory activity. Drugs without anti-inflammatory activity like phenelzine, chlorpromazine and desipramine, in spite of causing inhibition of Pg synthesis in vitro, failed to show any activity in vivo.

Despite the good correlation observed between anti-inflammatory activity and the effects of aspirin-like drugs on the spleen synthetase preparation, enzymes prepared from other tissues show different reactions to the drugs. On rabbit brain synthetase, for instance, the ratio of activity between indomethacin and aspirin is 17 : 1 (Flower and Vane, 1972), whereas on bovine seminal vesicles it is 2.140 : 1 (Ham et al., 1972). This important property, which may reflect a series of iso-enzymes, can explain the variations in activity within the group of compounds. For instance, the anti-pyretic analgesic drug 4-acetamidophenol (acetaminophen or paracetamol), which is 10 times less effective than aspirin on the dog spleen synthetase, has almost the same potency as aspirin on brain enzyme (Flower and Vane, 1972; Willis et al., 1972). Thus, the fact that para-cetamol has anti-pyretic activity without anti-inflammatory activity can be explained by the differential sensitivity of the prostaglandin synthetases from different tissues. Just as the anti-inflammatory activity of aspirin-like drugs correlates well with their action against spleen enzyme, so the anti-pyretic activity correlates with their action against the brain enzymes (Flower and Vane, 1972).

Other examples of differential enzyme sensitivity are also available. There is a thousand-fold variation in the ID_{50} of indomethacin against prostaglandin synthetases from different tissues of the rabbit (Bhattacherjee and Eakins, 1973). On the spleen enzyme, the ID_{50} was 0.05 $\mu g/ml$, and on the brain enzyme, 1.0 $\mu g/ml$ (these figures are in close agreement with those mentioned in the paper by Flower and Vane, 1972). On kidney enzyme, the ID_{50} was 5.0 $\mu g/ml$, on the iris ciliary body, 18.5 $\mu g/ml$ and on the retina 50 $\mu g/ml$.

One of the most important points in favour of the inhibition of the prosta-glandin biosynthesis as the mechanism of the anti-inflammatory action of aspirin-like drugs is that a therapeutic dose leads to a plasma concentration capable of causing a strong inhibition of the prostaglandin synthetases (Flower and Vane, 1972). Taking indomethacin as an example, the plasma concentration in man reaches 2 $\mu g/ml$. Because of protein binding (which is a property common to many of these drugs) the free plasma concentration would be 0.2 $\mu g/ml$. However, the ID_{50} for indomethacin on dog spleen synthetase is only 0.05 $\mu g/ml$. Hamberg (1972) calculated the daily prostaglandin turnover from the amounts of metabolites in the urine. Men consistently produced larger amounts (50–330 $\mu g/day$) than women (20–40 $\mu g/day$) but in both sexes there was a 77–98% inhibition of prostaglandin production by therapeutic doses of indometha-cin (200 mg daily), aspirin (3 g daily) or salicylate (3 g daily). Aspirin and its congeners at concentrations as low as those required to inhibit prostaglandin generation also block the release of a rabbit aorta contracting substance (RCS) from guinea pig lungs during anaphylaxis (Vargaftig and Dao, 1971; Piper and Vane, 1969). Several indications, including RCS formation from arachidonic acid (Vargaftig and Dao, 1971; Palmer et al., 1973), its appearance always with prostaglandins, its instability, and the inhibition of its release by aspirin-like drugs suggested to Gryglewski and Vane (1972) that RCS is the cyclic endoperoxide postulated as an unstable intermediate in the biosynthesis of prostaglandins. The cyclic endoperoxide was isolated and found to contract rabbit aorta (Hamberg and Samuelson, 1973). More recently, RCS was identi-fied as thromboxane, a new substance derived from oxidation of arachidonic acid which is capable of aggregating platelets and contracting rabbit aorta strips (Hamberg et al., 1975). If RCS is the cyclic endoperoxide or thromboxane, inhibition of its formation by aspirin-like drugs indicates an interference at an early stage of the synthesis of prostaglandins.

Generation of prostaglandin and inflammatory signs and symptoms

Cells do not store prostaglandins but have the capacity to synthesise and release them at the slightest provocation. Distortion of the cell membrane is a common thread between the different prostaglandin-producing stimuli which range through mechanical, pathological and chemical to physiological (Piper and Vane, 1971). Prostaglandins are generated in many forms of damage to the skin, both in animal and man, including carrageenan inflammation (Willis, 1969), contact dermatitis (Greaves et al., 1971) and inflammation due to ultra-violet light (Greaves and Søndergaard, 1970) and scalding (Änggård and Jonsson, 1971). The prostaglandin phase of carrageenan-induced paw swelling (Di Rosa et al., 1971a) as well as the increased concentration of prostaglandin in the carrageenan air bleb exudates were prevented by non-steroid anti-inflammatory drugs (Willis et al., 1972).

Detection of prostaglandins in biological fluids or inflammatory exudates depends upon the balance between generation by local (or migrating) cells and removal. The time at which prostaglandins reach detectable concentrations (2–3 hours; Willis, 1969) coincides with the arrival of polymorphonuclear cells (PMN) at the site of injury (Willis et al., 1972; Di Rosa et al., 1971b). As phagocytosis is accompanied by prostaglandin release (Higgs and Youlten, 1972), the continued presence of the injurious agent causes progressive increase of the prostaglandin concentration. Parallel to this, there is also a release of lysosomal enzymes which further damages the tissue (Willis et al., 1972). Another possible contribution of the lysosomal enzymes is to increase the local concentration of arachidonic acid by the action of phospholipase A upon plasma phospholipids, thus further increasing the generation of prostaglandins.

The importance of the PMN in the generation of prostaglandin is supported by the finding that: (a) up to 150 ng/ml of PGE can be detected in aqueous humour when it contains many PMN in experimental immunogenic uveitis in rabbits whereas the rabbit iris or ciliary body only generates $PGF_{2\alpha}$ (Eakins et al., 1972); (b) the appearance of prostaglandins in carrageenan air bleb exudates and the 'prostaglandin phase' of the carrageenan oedema parallel the migration of leucocytes (Willis et al., 1972; Di Rosa et al., 1971b); (c) certain immunosuppressive agents affect the 'prostaglandin phase' of the carrageenan oedema, by diminishing migration of PMN and monocytes (Van Arman and

Carlson, 1973). However, production of prostaglandins by the local cells must also be important since the early inflammatory reaction induced by carrageenan can be partially reduced by aspirin-like drugs.

We shall now discuss whether prostaglandin release can contribute to the genesis of fever, inflammation and pain, for if it can, then its abolition accounts for the anti-pyretic anti-inflammatory and analgesic actions of aspirin-like drugs.

Fever

Fever is often associated with an inflammatory process. Prostaglandin E_1 is the most powerful pyretic agent known, when injected either into cerebral ventricles or directly into the anterior hypothalamus (Milton and Wendlandt, 1971; Feldberg and Saxena, 1971). The hyperthermic effect is dose-dependent, almost immediate and lasts for about 3 hours. Prostaglandin E_1 causes fever by an action on the same region as that on which monoamines and pyrogens act to affect temperature. As in peripheral inflammatory responses, there is a generation of a prostaglandin E-like substance in the central nervous system during fever (Feldberg and Gupta, 1973) and the concentrations in the CSF rise after intravenous pyrogen by 2.5–4 times, sometimes to as much as 35 ng/ml.

Aspirin-like drugs do not abolish either the formation of endogenous pyrogen by leucocytes (Clark and Moyer, 1972) or the pyretic action of prostaglandins injected into the third ventricle of cats (Milton and Wendlandt, 1971). However, they inhibit both the generation of prostaglandins in the CNS and the fever caused by pyrogens of 5-hydroxytryptamine given into the cerebral ventricles. The 5- to 10-fold increase in prostaglandin release into the CSF observed at the height of endotoxin-induced fever in dogs was suppressed by the administration of indomethacin (Milton, 1973).

Pain

In man, prostaglandins cause pain along the veins into which they are infused and headache (Bergström et al., 1959; Collier et al., 1972). When administered intradermally (Ferreira, 1972) or intramuscularly (Karim, 1971) in concentrations much higher than those expected to occur in inflammation (Willis, 1969; Greaves and Søndergaard, 1970), prostaglandin E_1 causes a long-lasting overt pain. However, induction of hyperalgesia (i.e. a state in which pain can be elicited by normally painless mechanical or chemical stimulation) seems to be the typical effect of prostaglandins. Prostaglandins injected into dog knee joints produce incapacitation (Rosenthale et al., 1972), the reactions began within

15 minutes and lasted for several hours. Recently we have shown that prostaglandin but not histamine, bradykinin and 5-hydroxytryptamine acts together with the mediators released by carrageenan to produce hyperalgesia during the early phase of the inflammatory reaction in the rat paw (Ferreira et al., 1975b).

A long-lasting hyperalgesia was found when minute amounts of prostaglandin E_1 were given intradermally (Juhlin and Michaëlson, 1969) or infused subdermally (Ferreira, 1972). This hyperalgesia occurred with concentrations higher than those necessary to cause erythema. The subdermal infusion experiments, which were carried out in order to mimic the continuous release of mediators at the site of an injury, showed that the hyperalgesic effects of prostaglandins were cumulative, since they depended not only on their concentrations, but on the duration of the infusions. This cumulative sensitizing activity of the pain receptors was later also observed in dog's spleen (Ferreira et al., 1973) and rat paw (Willis and Cornelsen, 1973). In our experiments, during separate subdermal infusions of prostaglandin E_1, bradykinin or histamine (or a mixture of bradykinin and histamine) there was no overt pain; but when prostaglandin E_1 was added to bradykinin or histamine (or a mixture of both), strong pain occurred.

Another important observation concerned pruritus. Neither histamine, bradykinin nor prostaglandin E_1 infusions by themselves caused itching. However, when prostaglandin E_1 was infused with histamine, itching was always recorded (when prostaglandin E_1 was infused with bradykinin, there was pain rather than itching). This role of the prostaglandins in potentiating the effects of histamine has recently been confirmed (Greaves and McDonald-Gibson, 1973). The sensitizing action of prostaglandins to pain induced by bradykinin was shown to occur in the dog's spleen and knee joint also. Lim and his colleagues (Guzman et al., 1962, 1964; Lim et al., 1964) used nociception induced by intra-arterial injections of bradykinin into the spleen to show that aspirin-like drugs act peripherally as analgesics. To test whether bradykinin induces pain through prostaglandin release, we injected bradykinin into the spleen of the dog (Ferreira et al., 1973a, b). Prostaglandins were released in similar amounts, both in vitro and in vivo by injections of adrenaline or bradykinin. As adrenaline is a much weaker pain-producing substance than bradykinin in this system, it was clear that a prostaglandin could not be the *mediator* of the pain-producing activity of bradykinin.

In another series of experiments, we used the reflex rise in blood pressure induced by intra-arterial bradykinin injections into the spleen of lightly anaesthetized dogs as an indication of sensory stimulation. Doses of bradykinin which released prostaglandin from the spleen caused a reflex increase in blood pressure, in proportion to the dose used and these were reduced by indomethacin. When prostaglandin E_1 was given with the bradykinin in the indomethacin-treated dogs, the reflex increase in blood pressure was restored, sometimes to greater than control values (Ferreira et al., 1973a, b).

Extending this work, we have used the same technique to study the effect of prostaglandins on the nociceptive reflex induced by bradykinin injected into dog knee joints (Moncada et al., 1975). Increasing doses of bradykinin induced a dose-dependent rise in blood pressure. Local treatment with aspirin or indomethacin partially inhibited the bradykinin responses, probably by inhibiting the local formation of prostaglandins generated by the trauma caused by the manipulation of the joints. Infusion of prostaglandins produced a long-lasting potentiation of the algogenic effect of bradykinin. When local generation of prostaglandins was blocked by indomethacin and the enhanced sensitivity of the joints brought back by an infusion of prostaglandins, further injection of indomethacin did not alter the responses of the injection of bradykinin into the joints. This fact indicates that aspirin-like drugs do not affect the sensitivity of the receptors to the action of bradykinin.

At this stage we would like to return to RCS. RCS has strong pharmacological activity in that it contracts rabbit aorta and many other arterial muscle strips (Piper and Vane, 1969; Palmer et al., 1973) as do the lipoperoxides generated by lipoxidase acting on unsaturated fatty acids such as arachidonic, linoleic and linolenic acid (Gryglewski and Vane, 1972; Ferreira and Vargaftig, 1974). Thus, if RCS is a lipoperoxide intermediate in the formation of prostaglandins, it is possible that during prostaglandin biosynthesis, RCS can also contribute to the local pharmacological effects. Ferreira (1972) explored the possibility that fatty acid hydroperoxides can contribute to the genesis of pain in man. Intensity of the pain produced by intradermal injections of hydroperoxides of arachidonic, linoleic and linolenic acids was greater than that induced by either the parent fatty acids or acetylcholine, bradykinin, histamine or prostaglandin E_1. Recently (Hamberg et al., 1975), it was shown that another substance, thromboxane, generated by oxidation of arachidonic acid, which shares similarities with the endoperoxide intermediates of prostaglandin synthesis, causes contraction of rabbit aorta and platelet aggregation. The generation of this substance is also blocked by aspirin-like drugs. It was suggested that thromboxane can be identified as RCS.

From all these results we can make 3 conclusions: (1) Lipoperoxide intermediates in the prostaglandin biosynthetic pathway may have pain-producing properties, as do prostaglandin E_1 and E_2 in high concentrations; depending on the intensity of activation of the prostaglandin generating system by a trauma, the generation of the intermediate could exceed its conversion to prostaglandin, thus causing an acute type of pain. (2) In low concentrations, prostaglandin E_1 (and prostaglandin E_2) sensitize the pain fibres to mechanical and chemical stimuli. (3) The effects of prostaglandins E_1 and E_2 are cumulative and long-lasting. Thus, continual generation of minute amounts of prostaglandin at a site of injury will sensitize the nerves, so that mechanical stimulation or mediators such as bradykinin and histamine can cause pruritus or pain.

As we pointed out above, pain and fever are the first symptoms to be relieved during aspirin-like drug therapy. Later, there follows a diminution of the oedema and erythema. As already indicated, overt pain in an inflammatory reaction is probably a result of sensitization of the pain receptors to chemical or mechanical stimulation. The immediate relief of pain by drainage of an abscess illustrates the importance of the mechanical stimulus; however, during treatment with aspirin-like drugs the remission of pain due to inflammation of joints occurs before changes in the local amount of fluid. This may be due to the abolition of the sensitization of the pain receptors caused by prostaglandins. In support of this idea one may add that there is a dissociation between inflammatory oedema and hyperalgesia. Injection of dextran or passive cutaneous anaphylaxis cause a massive oedema without hyperalgesia. Addition of prostaglandins to these traumatic stimuli produced a much greater hyperalgesia than Pg alone. These results show that the inflammatory response depends on the balance of a number of mediators and the presence of hyperalgesia may indicate generation of prostaglandins (Ferreira et al., 1975b).

It is worth noting that aspirin-like drugs do not affect hyperalgesia or pain caused by direct action of prostaglandins. Aspirin, phenylbutazone or indomethacin were ineffective against the incapacitation induced by prostaglandins in the dog knee joint (Moncada et al., 1975). Indomethacin diminished the nociceptive effect of many agents injected intraperitoneally in mice (Thomas and West, 1973) or intra-arterially in dog spleen (Manjo et al., 1972; Crunkhorn and Willis, 1971), but it did not abolish either the writhing response in mice or the sensitization of dog's splenic sensory nerves induced by prostaglandins (Ferreira et al., 1973b; Thomas and West, 1973).

Thus, as in fever, the anti-inflammatory acids do not reduce the effects of prostaglandins but reduce those effects caused by substances which induce generation of prostaglandins. A possible exception to this is the action of *fenamates*, which have some antagonist action at receptors for prostaglandins (Collier and Sweatman, 1968) as well as potent anti-synthetase activity.

Erythema

Prostaglandins of the E and F series cause erythema in man and animals; prostaglandin E_1 is effective at doses as low as 1 ng; but for $F_{1\alpha}$ 1 μg is needed

(Juhlin and Michaëlson, 1969; Solomon et al., 1968). There are, however, two features of the vascular effects of prostaglandins not shared by other putative mediators of inflammation. The first is a sustained action and the second is the ability to counteract the vasoconstriction caused by substances such as noradrenaline and angiotensin. The erythema induced by intradermal injection or subdermal infusions (Ferreira, 1972) illustrates well the long-lasting action of prostaglandins (sometimes up to 10 hours). This confers a very important property upon the prostaglandins, in that the appearance and the magnitude of their effects not only depend on the actual concentration but also upon the duration of their release of infusion (Ferreira, 1972).

Oedema

Prostaglandins, like bradykinin, histamine and 5-hydroxytryptamine, cause increased vascular permeability by inducing vascular linkage at the post-capillary and collecting venules (Kaley and Weiner, 1971). Although most active substances exhibit a general relationship between ability to increase vascular permeability and erythema formation, these effects result from actions on different components of the vessel. Erythema represents a local pooling of blood due to a relaxation of the smooth muscles of the walls of arterioles and venules, whereas increased vascular permeability is now thought to result from the contraction of the venular endothelial cells (Majno et al., 1972). In fact, prostaglandins produce vasodilation more effectively than oedema. Prostaglandin E_1 when compared with histamine in the guinea pig skin, produces an equivalent and much longer lasting erythema but a smaller wheal (Solomon et al., 1968). Similarly, in man, histamine, bradykinin and prostaglandin E_1 each cause erythema and oedema when injected intradermally. However, prostaglandin E_1 induces long-lasting erythema and a much less pronounced oedema (Ferreira, 1972). There is no difference in the duration of the increased vascular permeability induced in rats by histamine or prostaglandin (Crunkhorn and Willis, 1971).

Prostaglandins E_1, E_2 and A_2 but not $F_{2\alpha}$ caused oedema when injected into the hind paws of rats (Glenn et al., 1972). Prostaglandin E_1 (on a weight basis) was as effective as bradykinin, though higher doses (40–80 μg), instead of causing increased effects like bradykinin, produced erythema without oedema. When prostaglandin E_1 was given together with histamine or 5-hydroxytryptamine, it elicited an additive effect rather than a synergistic one. However, it is possible that in these experiments, endogenous prostaglandins were produced by the trauma of the injection and that these contributed to the resultant oedema. To avoid such a possibility, we treated rats with indomethacin to prevent endogenous formation of prostaglandins (Moncada et al., 1973; Ferreira et al., 1974). This reduced the paw oedema produced by bradykinin and by prostaglandin E_1, given separately, but had no effect on oedema produced by the combination of the two. Thus, the injection itself, or the events which follow it, can cause prostaglandin release which will increase the effects of the injected substance. When endogenous prostaglandin release is prevented by indomethacin, there is a clear synergism between the effects of bradykinin and prostaglandin E_1. Thomas and West (1973) also studied the effects of prostaglandins or 5-hydroxytryptamine on the permeability increase in rat skin induced by bradykinin. They found that small doses of PGE_1 selectively potentiated bradykinin. In rabbit, PGE_2 also enhanced the increase in permeability induced by bradykinin (Harrison, 1973).

If a prostaglandin is sensitizing blood vessels to the permeability effects of other mediators (as happens with pain receptors), then the actions of anti-inflammatory drugs on oedema can be explained by removal of this sensitization. Thus, the contribution which prostaglandins make to the oedema of inflammation is by increasing the effect of the other known mediators, such as histamine and bradykinin. To test this idea, carrageenan-induced paw swelling was measured in rats treated with indomethacin. Low concentrations of prostaglandin E_1 added to the carrageenan injection strikingly increased the oedema formation. Clearly, prostaglandin E_1 can sensitize the blood vessels to the permeability increasing effects of the other mediators locally released by carrageenan and removal of endogenous prostaglandin generation (and therefore of the sensitization) explains the anti-oedema effects of aspirin-like drugs (Moncada et al., 1973).

References

ÄNGGÅRD, E. and JONSSON, C. E. (1971): *Acta physiol. scand.*, *81*, 440.

BERGSTRÖM, S., DUNER, H., VON EULER, U. S., PERNOW, B. and SJOVALL, J. (1959): *Acta physiol. scand.*, *45*, 145.

BHATTACHERJEE, P. and EAKINS, K. E. (1973): *Pharmacologist*, *15*, 209.

CHANG, Y. H. (1972): *J. Pharmacol. exp. Ther.*, *183*, 235.

CLARK, W. G. and MOYER, S. G. (1972): *J. Pharmacol. exp. Ther.*, *181*, 183.

COLLIER, H. O. J. and SCHNEIDER, C. (1972): *Nature New Biol.*, *236*, 141.

COLLIER, H. O. J. and SWEATMAN, W. J. F. (1968): *Nature (Lond.)*, *219*, 864.

COLLIER, J. G., KARIM, S. M. M., ROBINSON, B. and SOMERS, K. (1972): *Brit. J. Pharmacol.*, *44*, 374.

CRUNKHORN, P. and WILLIS, A. L. (1971): *Brit. J. Pharmacol.*, *41*, 49.

DI ROSA, M., GIROUD, J. P. and WILLOUGHBY, D. A. (1971a): *J. Path.*, *104*, 15.

DI ROSA, M., PAPADIMITRIOU, J. M. and WILLOUGHBY, D. A. (1971b): *J. Path.*, *105*, 239.

EAKINS, K. E., WHITELOCK, R. I. F., PERKINS, E. S., BENNETT, A. and UNGAR, W. G. (1972): *Nature New Biol.*, *239*, 248.

FELDBERG, W. and GUPTA, K. P. (1973): *J. Physiol. (Lond.)*, *228*, 41.

FELDBERG, W. and SAXENA, P. N. (1971): *J. Physiol. (Lond.)*, *217*, 547.

FERREIRA, S. H. (1972): *Nature New Biol.*, *240*, 200.

FERREIRA, S. H., HARVEY, A., HIGGS, G. A. and VANE, J. R. (1975a): In: *Abstracts, International Conference on Prostaglandins, Florence*, p. 40.

FERREIRA, S. H., HARVEY, E. A. and VANE, J. R. (1975b): In: *Abstracts, VI International Congress of Pharmacology, Helsinki*, Abstr. No. 1001.

FERREIRA, S. H., MONCADA, S. and VANE, J. R. (1971): *Nature New Biol.*, *231*, 237.

FERREIRA, S. H., MONCADA, S. and VANE, J. R. (1973a): *Brit. J. Pharmacol.*, *47*, 48.

FERREIRA, S. H., MONCADA, S. and VANE, J. R. (1973b): *Brit. J. Pharmacol.*, *49*, 86.

FERREIRA, S. H., MONCADA, S. and VANE, J. R. (1974): In: *Prostaglandin Synthetase Inhibitors*, pp. 175–187. Editors: H. J. Robinson and J. R. Vane. Raven Press, New York.

FERREIRA, S. H. and VANE, J. R. (1974a): *Ann. Rev. Pharmacol.*, *14*, 57.

FERREIRA, S. H. and VANE, J. R. (1974b): In: *The Prostaglandins, II*, pp. 1–39. Editor: P. W. Ramwell. Plenum Press, New York–London.

FERREIRA, S. H. and VARGAFTIG, B. B. (1974): *Brit. J. Pharmacol.*, *50*, 543.

FLOWER, R. J. and CHEUNG, H. S. (1973): *Prostaglandins*, *4*, 325.

FLOWER, R. J., GRYGLEWSKI, R., HERBACZYNSKA, C. K. and VANE, J. R. (1972): *Nature New Biol.*, *238*, 107.

FLOWER, R. J. and VANE, J. R. (1972): *Nature (Lond.)*, *240*, 410.

GLENN, E. M., BOWMAN, B. J. and ROHLOFF, N. A. (1972): In: *Prostaglandins in Cellular Biology*, p. 329. Editors: P. W. Ramwell and B. P. Pharris. Plenum Press, New York-London.

GREAVES, M. W. and MCDONALD-GIBSON, W. (1973): *Brit. med. J.*, *3*, 308.

GREAVES, M. W. and SØNDERGAARD, J. (1970): *J. invest. Derm.*, *54*, 365.

GREAVES, M. W., SØNDERGAARD, J. and MCDONALD-GIBSON, W. (1971): *Brit. med. J.*, *2*, 258.

GRYGLEWSKI, R. and VANE, J. R. (1972): *Brit. J. Pharmacol.*, *45*, 37.

GUZMAN, F., BRAUN, C. and LIM, R. K. S. (1962): *Arch. int. Pharmacodyn.*, *136*, 353.

GUZMAN, F., BRAUN, C., LIM, R. K. S., POTTER, G. D. and RODGERS, D. W. (1964): *Arch. int. Pharmacodyn.*, *149*, 571.

HAM, E. A., CIRILLO, V. J., ZANETTI, M., SHEN, T. Y. and KUEHL JR, F. A. (1972): In: *Prostaglandins in Cellular Biology*, pp. 343–352. Editors: P. W. Ramwell and B. P. Pharris. Plenum Press, New York–London.

HAMBERG, M. (1972): *Biochem. biophys. Res. Commun.*, *49*, 720.

HAMBERG, M. and SAMUELSSON, B. (1973): *Proc. nat. Acad. Sci. (Wash.)*, *70*, 899.

HAMBERG, M., SVENSSON, J. and SAMUELSSON, B. (1975): In: *Proceedings, International Conference on Prostaglandins, Florence*, p. 3.

HARRISON, R. G. (1973): *Int. Res. Commun. System, June 1973 (8–11–2)*.

HIGGS, G. A. and YOULTEN, L. J. F. (1972): *Brit. J. Pharmacol.*, *44*, 330.

JUHLIN, S. and MICHAËLSON, G. (1969): *Acta derm.-venereol. (Stockh.)*, *49*, 251.

KALEY, G. and WEINER, R. (1971): *Ann. N.Y. Acad. Sci.*, *180*, 338.

KARIM, S. M. M. (1971): *Ann. N.Y. Acad. Sci.*, *180*, 483.

LIM, R. K. S., GUZMAN, F., RODGERS, D. W., GOTO, K., BRAUN, G., DICKERSON, D. G. and ENGLE, R. J. (1964): *Arch. int. Pharmacodyn.*, *152*, 25.

MAJNO, G., RYAN, G. B., GABBIANI, G., HIRSCHEL, B. J., IRLE, C. and JORIS, I. (1972): In: *Inflammation, Mechanisms and Control*, pp. 13–39. Editors: Irwin H. Lepow and Peter Ward. Academic Press, New York–London.

MILTON, A. S. (1973): In: *Proceedings, International Conference on Prostaglandins, Vienna,* pp. 495–500. Pergamon Press-Vieweg, Braunschweig.

MILTON, A. S. and WENDLANDT, S. (1971): *J. Physiol. (Lond.), 218,* 325.

MONCADA, S., FERREIRA, S. H. and VANE, J. R. (1973): *Nature (Lond.), 246,* 217.

MONCADA, S., FERREIRA, S. H. and VANE, J. R. (1975): *Europ. J. Pharmacol., 31,* 250.

PALMER, M. A., PIPER, P. J. and VANE, J. R. (1973): *Brit. J. Pharmacol., 49,* 226.

PIPER, P. J. and VANE, J. R. (1969): In: *Prostaglandins, Peptides and Amines,* pp. 15–19. Editors: P. Montegazza and E. W. Horton. Academic Press, London–New York.

PIPER, P. J. and VANE, J. R. (1971): *Ann. N. Y. Acad. Sci., 180,* 363.

ROSENTHALE, M. E., DERVINIS, A., KASSARICH, J. and SINGER, S. (1972): *J. Pharm. Pharmacol., 24,* 149.

SMITH, J. B. and WILLIS, A. L. (1971): *Nature New Biol., 231,* 235.

SMITH, M. J. and DAWKINS, P. D. (1971): *J. Pharm. Pharmacol., 23,* 729.

SOLOMON, L. M., JUHLIN, L. and KIRSCHENBAUM, M. B. (1968): *J. invest. Derm., 51,* 280.

TAKEGUCHI, C. and SIH, C. J. (1972): *Prostaglandins, 2,* 169.

THOMAS, G. and WEST, G. B. (1973): *J. Pharm. Pharmacol., 25,* 747.

TOMLINSON, R. V., RINGOLD, H. J., QURESHI, M. C. and FORCHIELLI, E. (1972): *Biochem. biophys. Res. Commun., 46,* 552.

VAN ARMAN, C. G. and CARLSON, R. P. (1973): In: *Future Trends in Inflammation,* pp. 159–169. Editors: G. P. Velo, D. A. Willoughby and J. P. Giroud. Piccin Medical Books, Padua and London.

VANE, J. R. (1971): *Nature New Biol., 231,* 232.

VARGAFTIG, B. P. and DAO, N. (1971): *Pharmacology, 6,* 99.

WILLIS, A. L. (1969): In: *Prostaglandins, Peptides and Amines,* pp. 31–38. Editors: P. Montegazza and E. W. Horton. Academic Press, London–New York.

WILLIS, A. L. and CORNELSEN, M. (1973): *Prostaglandins, 3,* 353.

WILLIS, A. L., DAVIDSON, P., RAMWELL, P. W., BROCKLEBURST, W. E. and SMITH, B. (1972): In: *Prostaglandins in Cellular Biology,* pp. 227–259. Editors: P. W. Ramwell and B. P. Pharris. Plenum Press, New York–London.

Platelets, inflammation and non-steroidal anti-inflammatory drugs

Giovanni de Gaetano

Laboratorio Ricerche sulla Emostasi e Trombosi, Istituto di Ricerche Farmacologiche 'Mario Negri', Milan, Italy

Platelets have been recognized for many years as playing a fundamental role in haemostasis and in the pathogenesis of thrombosis (see for reviews Vermylen et al., 1973; Mustard and Packham, 1975; de Gaetano et al., 1975; Walsh, 1975). More recently, evidence has been accumulated to support a relationship between haemostasis and the inflammatory process, with platelets being the main link between these two phenomena (see for review Silver et al., 1974b).

If one considers inflammation as a local reaction to injury of the living microcirculation and its contents (Spector and Willoughby, 1968), then the haemostatic process can be considered as a form of inflammation. Both the haemostatic and inflammatory processes may be triggered by the same pathological events and occur almost simultaneously.

Within a few seconds of a blood vessel being injured, platelets adhere to subendothelial tissue (collagen, microfibrils, Willebrand factor) and to each other; the latter phenomenon is called 'aggregation' and is mediated by the local availability of adenosine-5'-diphosphate (ADP) released from adhering platelets.

The release of endogenous ADP is accompanied by the release of several other biologically active substances, a phenomenon known as the 'release reaction' (Holmsen et al., 1969). They include serotonin, prostaglandins E_2 and $F_{2\alpha}$, hydrolytic enzymes including phospholipase A_1, heparin neutralizing activity, cationic proteins and a factor stimulating the growth of cultured vascular smooth muscle cells.

Serotonin seems not to play an important role in haemostasis since the bleeding time is not prolonged in man (Haverbach et al., 1957) or in rats (Wielosz et al., 1976) that have been reserpinized and whose platelets are devoid of serotonin. On the other hand, serotonin is known to cause vasoconstriction, to increase vascular permeability and to produce or potentiate fever (Zucker, 1947; Majno et al., 1967; Myers, 1911).

PGE_2 is produced in relatively large amounts by platelets during platelet aggregation or blood clotting (Smith and Willis, 1971; Silver et al., 1972; Smith et al., 1973a). PGE_2 increases vascular permeability, potentiates increased vascular permeability caused by histamine or bradykinin, increases blood flow, produces or potentiates pain and fever, enhances chemotaxis, causes experimental arthritis and potentiates carrageenan-induced rat paw swelling. In addition, PGE_2 has been found in the exudates from carrageenan-induced oedema in the rat paw and in human burn blister fluid (for detailed references, see Silver et al., 1974a).

PGE_2 (and $PGF_{2\alpha}$) are synthesized by platelets from arachidonic acid (Silver et al., 1973; Vargaftig and Zirinis, 1973). More recently, it has been shown that aggregating agents such as ADP activate phospholipase in the platelet membrane, releasing arachidonic acid and possibly triggering the sequence of reactions leading to prostaglandin synthesis (Smith et al., 1973b; Schoene and Iacono, 1975). During prostaglandin formation in the platelets, one or more cyclic endoperoxide intermediates transiently accumulate in the cell and are capable of inducing the release reaction and platelet aggregation (Smith et al., 1974; Hamberg and Samuelsson, 1974; Hamberg et al., 1974; Willis, 1974). PGE_2 (and to a much lesser extent $PGF_{2\alpha}$) sensitize platelets to the aggregating activity of endoperoxides (Willis, 1974), which explains the previously observed potentiation of irreversible aggregation and release reaction induced by PGE_2 (Kloeze, 1969). Intravenous injection of arachidonate or of endoperoxides into experimental animals is followed by rapid death associated with intravascular platelet aggregates (Willis, 1974; Silver et al., 1974a). It has also been shown recently that some of the biologically active substances formed by platelets from arachidonate cause contraction of rabbit aorta (Vargaftig and Zirinis, 1973).

Besides PGE_2, other factors which increase vascular permeability may be released from stimulated platelets, a phenomenon first observed by Mustard et al. (1965). One of these is a cationic protein of about 30,000 mol. wt. reported by Nachman et al. (1972).

More recently, platelets have been found to be a source of fibroblast growth-promoting activity (Kohler and Lipton, 1974) and of a factor stimulating the proliferation of arterial smooth-muscle cells (Ross et al., 1974). In this regard the observation that human fibroblasts, like platelets, are able to induce fibrin retraction (Niewiarowski et al., 1972; Dolfini et al., 1976) is of interest.

The ingestion of therapeutic amounts of aspirin in man results in a definite prolongation of the bleeding time (see de Gaetano et al., 1975) and a marked inhibition of platelet aggregation and of the release of nucleotides and serotonin from platelets (see Mustard and Packham, 1975). The frequent haemorrhagic side effects of treatment with aspirin may result for a great part from these properties (see de Gaetano et al., 1975).

In 1971 Smith and Willis showed that platelet biosynthesis of prostaglandins induced by thrombin stimulation was markedly inhibited by aspirin and indomethacin after oral ingestion in small doses. Sodium salicylate had only a weak effect; phenylbutazone had an activity intermediate between aspirin and sodium salicylate, whereas acetaminophen (paracetamol) and cortisone were inactive. To a remarkable degree these results reflect the relative ability of these drugs to suppress release reaction and irreversible aggregation (O'Brien, 1968; Zucker and Peterson, 1970). Subsequently, Kocsis et al. (1973) have shown that, after oral administration of aspirin or indomethacin to human subjects, the duration of the inhibitory effects of both drugs on platelet prostaglandin production parallels their effects on platelet release reaction and aggregation (several days or a few hours, respectively) (O'Brien et al., 1970; de Gaetano et al., 1971).

The inhibitory action of aspirin on platelet aggregation could be prevented by arachidonic acid, an observation which led to the suggestion that some arachidonate-consuming processes would be involved in platelet release and aggregation (Leonardi et al., 1973). This hypothesis received strong support from the finding that an acetylenic analog (TYA) of arachidonic acid inhibits, like aspirin, both prostaglandin formation and platelet aggregation (Willis et al., 1974). The biosynthesis of pro-aggregatory endoperoxide intermediates is also blocked by aspirin or TYA. Possibly aspirin and related drugs inhibit the platelet prostaglandin synthetases, whereas TYA competes with the substrate in arachidonate-utilizing enzyme systems (Willis et al., 1974).

The new light recently cast on the complex mechanisms of platelet aggregation justifies the remarkable effort presently being made to evaluate whether drugs that interfere with prostaglandin biosynthesis have clinical value as antithrombotic drugs. This subject has been extensively covered by recent reviews (Vermylen et al., 1973; Didisheim et al., 1974; Hirsh et al., 1975; Mustard and Packham, 1975). Substantial evidence has already been found to suggest that aspirin and other non-steroidal anti-inflammatory drugs may be beneficial in the management of coronary and cerebrovascular atherosclerosis and in venous thromboembolism.

Indomethacin has been shown to reduce intravascular fibrin deposition and the urinary excretion of fibrinogen-related material in patients affected by chronic glomerulonephritis (Vermylen et al., 1970; Clarkson et al., 1972; de Gaetano et al., 1974).

In conclusion, platelets play a crucial role in haemostasis and thrombosis and may well play an equally relevant role in inflammation. Platelets were found in small blood vessels or enmeshed in fibrin at inflammation sites (Cotran, 1965; McKay, 1972) and were both quantitatively and qualitatively altered in the blood of rats a few hours after initiating carrageenan pleurisy (Zawilska et al., 1973) and during the early development of adjuvant-induced arthritis (Lassman et al., 1974). On the other hand, the active Arthus reaction did not occur in thrombocytopenic animals (Margaretten and McKay, 1971). The fact that non-steroidal anti-inflammatory drugs are also anti-haemostatic and anti-thrombotic agents makes it possible that the anti-inflammatory activity of these drugs resides to a degree in their ability to interfere specifically with the formation and release of inflammatory substances from platelets (O'Brien, 1968; Silver et al., 1974b).

Acknowledgements

I thank Dr. Melvin J. Silver, Cardeza Foundation and Department of Pharmacology, Thomas Jefferson University, Philadelphia, Pa., U.S.A. for drawing my attention to several works referred to in this review. Mrs. Amy Crook, Miss Paola Bonifacino and Miss Anna Mancini gave valuable help in the preparation of this manuscript.

References

CLARKSON, A. R., MacDONALD, M. K., CASH, J. D. and ROBSON, J. S. (1972): Modification by drugs of urinary fibrin/fibrinogen degradation products in glomerulonephritis. *Brit. med. J.*, *3*, 255.

COTRAN, R. S. (1965): The delayed and prolonged vascular leakage inflammation II. An electron microscopic study of the vascular response after thermal injury. *Amer. J. Path.*, *46*, 589.

DE GAETANO, G., DONATI, M. B. and GARATTINI, S. (1975): Drugs affecting platelet function tests. Their effects on haemostasis and surgical bleeding. *Thrombos. Diathes. haemorrh. (Stuttg.)*, *34*, 285.

DE GAETANO, G., DONATI, M. B. and VERMYLEN, J. (1971): Some effects of indomethacin on platelet function, blood coagulation and fibrinolysis. *Int. Z. klin. Pharmakol. Ther. Toxikol.*, 2, 196.

DE GAETANO, G., VERMYLEN, J., DONATI, M. B., DOTREMONT, G. and MICHIELSEN, P. (1974): Indomethacin and platelet aggregation in chronic glomerulonephritis: existence of non-responders. *Brit. med. J.*, 2, 301.

DIDISHEIM, P., KAZMIER, F. J. and FUSTER, V. (1974): Platelet inhibition in the management of thrombosis. *Thrombos. Diathes. haemorrh. (Stuttg.)*, 32, 21.

DOLFINI, E., AZZARONE, B., DONATI, M. B., DE GAETANO, G., OTTAVIANO, E. and MORASCA, L. (1976): Attività piastrino-simile di cellule animali ed umane in coltura. In: *Atti del Congresso Società Italiana di Microbiologia, Padova, Italia, Ottobre 1975*, in press.

HAMBERG, M. and SAMUELSSON, B. (1974): Prostaglandin endoperoxides. Novel transformations of arachidonic acid in human platelets. *Proc. nat. Acad. Sci. (Wash.)*, 71, 3400.

HAMBERG, M., SVENSSON, J., WAKABAYASHI, T. and SAMUELSSON, B. (1974): Isolation and structure of two prostaglandin endoperoxides that cause platelet aggregation. *Proc. nat. Acad. Sci. (Wash.)*, 71, 345.

HAVERBACK, B. J., DUTCHER, T. F., SHORE, P. A., TOMICH, E. G., TERRY, L. L. and BRODIE, B. B. (1957): Serotonin changes in platelets and brain induced by small daily doses of reserpine. Lack of effect of depletion of platelet serotonin on hemostatic mechanisms. *New Engl. J. Med.*, 256, 343.

HIRSH, J., GENT, M. and GENTON, E. (1975): The current status of platelet suppressive drugs in the treatment of thrombosis. *Thrombos. Diathes. haemorrh. (Stuttg.)*, 33, 406.

HOLMSEN, H., DAY, H. J. and STORMORKEN, H. (1969): The blood platelet release reaction. *Scand. J. Haemat., Suppl. 8*, 3.

KLOEZE, J. (1969): Relationship between chemical structure and platelet-aggregation activity of prostaglandins. *Biochim. biophys. Acta (Amst.)*, 187, 285.

KOCSIS, J. J., HERNANDOVICH, J., SILVER, M. J., SMITH, J. B. and INGERMAN, C. (1973): Duration of inhibition of platelet prostaglandin formation and aggregation by ingested aspirin or indomethacin. *Prostaglandins 3*, 141.

KOHLER, N. and LIPTON, A. (1971): Platelets as a source of fibroblast growth-promoting activity. *Exp. Cell Res.*, 87, 297.

LASSMAN, H. B., KIRBY, R. E. and NOVICK JR., W. J. (1974): Alterations in platelet aggregation associated with adjuvant arthritis in rats. *Pharmacol. Res. Commun.*, 6, 493.

LEONARDI, R. G., ALEXANDER, B. and WHITE, F. (1973): Prevention of aspirin inhibition of platelet release reaction by the fatty acid precursor of platelet prostaglandins. *Thromb. Res.*, 3, 327.

MAJNO, G., GILMORE, V. and LEVENTHAL, M. (1967): On the mechanism of vascular leakage caused by histamine-type mediators. A microscopic study in vivo. *Circ. Res.*, 21, 833.

MARGARETTEN, W. and MCKAY, D. G. (1971): The requirement for platelets in the active arthus reaction. *Amer. J. Path.*, 64, 257.

MCKAY, D. G. (1972): Participation of components of the blood coagulation system in the inflammatory response. *Amer. J. Path.*, 67, 181.

MUSTARD, J. F., MOVAT, H. Z., MACMORINE, D. R. L. and SENYI, A. (1965): Release of permeability factors from the blood platelet. *Proc. Soc. exp. Biol. (N.Y.)*, 119, 988.

MUSTARD, J. F. and PACKHAM, M. A. (1975): Platelets, thrombosis and drugs. *Drugs*, 9, 19.

MYERS, R. D. (1911): Hypothalamic mechanisms of pyrogen action in the cat and monkey. In: *Pyrogens and Fever*. Editors: G. E. W. Wolstenholme and J. Birch. Churchill Livingstone, Edinburgh.

NACHMAN, R. L., WEKSLER, B. and FERRIS, B. (1972): Characterization of human platelet vascular permeability-enhancing activity. *J. clin. Invest.*, *51*, 549.

NIEWIAROWSKI, S., REGOECZI, E. and MUSTARD, J. F. (1972): Adhesion of fibroblasts to polymerizing fibrin and retraction of fibrin induced by fibroblasts. *Proc. Soc. exp. Biol. (N.Y.)*, *140*, 199.

O'BRIEN, J. R. (1968): Effect of anti-inflammatory agents on platelets. *Lancet*, *1*, 894.

O'BRIEN, J. R., FINCH, W. and CLARK, E. (1970): A comparison of an effect of different anti-inflammatory drugs on human platelets. *J. clin. Path.*, *23*, 522.

ROSS, R., GLOMSET, J., KARIYA, B. and HARKER, L. (1974): A platelet-dependent serum factor that stimulates the proliferation of arterial smooth muscle Cells 'in vitro'. *Proc. nat. Acad. Sci. (Wash.)*, *71*, 1207.

SCHOENE, N. W. and IACONO, J. M. (1975): Stimulation of platelet phospholipase A_2 activity by aggregating agents. *Fed. Proc.*, *34*, 257.

SILVER, M. J., HOCH, W., KOCSIS, J. J., INGERMAN, C. M. and SMITH, J. B. (1974a): Arachidonic acid causes sudden death in rabbits. *Science*, *183*, 1085.

SILVER, M. J., SMITH, J. B. and INGERMAN, C. M. (1974b): Blood platelets and the inflammatory process. *Agents Actions*, *4*, 233.

SILVER, M. J., SMITH, J. B., INGERMAN, C. and KOCSIS, J. J. (1972): Human blood prostaglandins; formation during clotting. *Prostaglandins*, *1*, 429.

SILVER, M. J., SMITH, J. B., INGERMAN, C. and KOCSIS, J. J. (1973): Arachidonic acid-induced human platelet aggregation and prostaglandin formation. *Prostaglandins*, *4*, 863.

SMITH, J. B., INGERMAN, C., KOCSIS, J. J. and SILVER, M. J. (1973a): Formation of prostaglandins during the aggregation of human blood platelets. *J. clin. Invest.*, *52*, 965.

SMITH, J. B., INGERMAN, C., KOCSIS, J. J. and SILVER, M. J. (1974): Formation of an intermediate in prostaglandin biosynthesis and its association with the platelet release reaction. *J. clin. Invest.*, *53*, 1468.

SMITH, J. B., SILVER, M. J. and WEBSTER, G. R. (1973b): Phospholipase A_1 of human blood platelets. *Biochem. J.*, *131*, 615.

SMITH, J. B. and WILLIS, A. L. (1971): Aspirin selectively inhibits prostaglandin production in human platelets. *Nature New Biol.*, *231*, 235.

SPECTOR, W. G. and WILLOUGHBY, D. A. (1968): *The Pharmacology of Inflammation*. English Universities Press, London.

VARGAFTIG, B. B. and ZIRINIS, P. (1973): Platelet aggregation induced by arachidonic acid is accompanied by release of potential inflammatory mediators distinct from PGE_2 and PGF_{2a}. *Nature new Biol.*, *244*, 114.

VERMYLEN, J., DE GAETANO, G. and VERSTRAETE, M. (1973): Platelets and thrombosis. In: *Recent Advances in Thrombosis*, p. 113. Editor: L. Poller. Churchill Livingstone, Edinburgh.

VERMYLEN, J., DOTREMONT, G., DE GAETANO, G., DONATI, M. B. and MICHIELSEN, P. (1970): Indomethacin and urinary excretion of fibrinogen-like material in proliferative glomerulonephritis. *Rev. Eur. Étud. clin. biol.*, *15*, 979.

WALSH, P. N. (1975): The possible role of platelet coagulant activities in the pathogenesis of venous thrombosis. *Thrombos. Diathes. haemorrh. (Stuttg.)*, *33*, 435.

WIELOSZ, M., STELLA, L. and DE GAETANO, G. (1976): Bleeding time in laboratory animals II. Lack of effect of depletion of platelet serotonin in rat. *Thromb. Res.*, submitted for publication.

WILLIS, A. L. (1974): Isolation of a chemical trigger for thrombosis. *Prostaglandins*, *5*, 1.

WILLIS, A. L., KUHN, D. C. and WEISS, H. J. (1974): Acetylenic analog of arachidonate that acts like aspirin on platelets. *Science*, *183*, 327.

ZAWILSKA, K., GIROUD, J. P., TIMSIT, J. and CAEN, J. P. (1973): Plaquettes et inflammation. I. Etude chez le rat des variations quantitatives et qualitatives des plaquettes au cours d'une réaction inflammatoire aigue (pleurésis à la carragénine). *Path. Biol.*, *21*, *Suppl.*, 51.

ZUCKER, M. B. (1947): Platelet agglutination and vasoconstriction as factors in spontaneous hemostasis in normal, thrombocytopenic, heparinized and hypoprothrombinemic rats. *Amer. J. Physiol.*, *148*, 275.

ZUCKER, M. B. and PETERSON, J. (1970): Effect of acetylsalicyclic acid, other nonsteroidal anti-inflammatory agents, and dipyridamole on human blood platelets. *J. Lab. clin. Med.*, *76*, 66.

Complement and inflammation: an approach to the pharmacology of the complement system*

T. di Perri and A. Auteri

Istituto di Semeiotica Medica, University of Siena, Italy

The serum complement system is made up of nine proteic components identified as C1–C9. The first is called C1 and is idvided into three subfractions – C1q, C1r, C1s – which interact to form C1 activated in response to any specific stimulation. So, really, there are twelve components.

The different components of the complement system have been well characterised from both the physical and chemical point of view, and all of them have been extracted and purified from serum. By the use of classic methods, it has been possible to prepare monospecific antisera for each component. These antisera have been particularly useful in achieving standard elective methods of dosage and identification.

The serum complement system must play a particular role in the homeostatic control of the human body. Some difficulties have arisen in the definition of the physiologic role of the complement system, since some of the mechanisms are not entirely understood and have not been observed under pathologic conditions, either experimentally or clinically. However, it should be underlined that it is particularly difficult to clearly distinguish between physiology and pathology each time we have a possible impairment of an homeostatic mechanism. On the other hand, the whole phenomenon might be evaluated in a different way. These considerations do not lessen the problem, but only stress that our physio-

* Supported by a Research Grant (No. 709) from OTAN, Brussels.

pathologic knowledge of complement is not so advanced that we clearly understand its functional activity.

Another problem, which is particularly topical, concerns the widespread opinion that the complement system is an inseparable functional entity, while it appears to be more and more clear that the single components have their own specific functions which may be active outside the usual system, even though all these components cooperate in the activation of the whole complement system. These specific functions of some components of the complement system are responsible for a mono- or bidirectional control of the activation of other proteic systems which appear to be functionally correlated, such as the coagulation system, fibrinolysis and kinin-forming system. They also participate in the biological release of the chemical mediators of inflammation and the functional activities of the inflammatory cells, such as leukocyte and platelet chemotaxis, leukocyte degranulation and platelet aggregation.

This functional profile shows how closely the complement system is involved in the acute inflammatory process. But recent data underline that at least one component of the complement system, the C3 fraction, is particularly active in the immunological regulation of inflammation, especially as regards antibody synthesis and immune complex production (Dukor et al., 1974). It has been shown that the in vitro activation of the C3 fraction by the alternative pathway induced by cobra venom factor may be a functional substitute for T lymphocytes in T-dependent antibody synthesis. Dukor and Hartman (1973) and Bokisch et al. (1969) reported that a subfraction of component C3, C3b, has mitogen properties for B lymphocytes. Dukor and Hartman (1973) advanced the hypothesis that the products deriving from the splitting of the C3 component may represent a second non-specific activation of B lymphocytes, interacting with those lymphocytes which bring on their membrane complement receptors.

Pepys and Butterworth (1974) have been able to show that C3 depletion induced by cobra venom factor causes a selective depression of the T-dependent antibody response, while the T-independent response seems to be unaffected. Dukor et al. (1974) arrived at the same conclusion using different methods of investigation. So it may be suggested, following Feldmann and Pepys (1974), that the C3 fraction may mediate the adhesion process of the complexes between antigen and T cell carriers of immunoglobulins to the macrophages, thus improving the efficacy of the antigenic activity to the B cell.

A particular role in this field is probably played by C3a, another product of C3 splitting, which should be responsible for mediator release from macrophages. Dukor et al. (1974) hypothesised that C3a may be produced by T-dependent antigens and B cell mitogens in the presence of complement to stimulate the release of B lymphocyte-activating factors from macrophages.

On the other hand, T-dependent antigens react first of all against T cells, which produce a complement activation factor giving rise to C3a and then the release from macrophages of stimulating factors which finally activate B cells.

It is particularly interesting that in both situations the inhibition of C3 activation may cause a selective block of B-cell activation in favour of differentiation into antibody-producing cells (Dukor et al., 1974).

C3 fraction has been shown to stimulate the linkage between B cells and antigen-antibody complexes or B cells and aggregated IgG, as reported in some experimental work (Dukor et al., 1974). Probably the C3 fraction is also the modulator of the B cell carrier function of the antigen toward the germinal centers of lymph nodes, and of the localisation of lymphocytes with membrane receptors for C3 in lymphoid follicles (Bianco et al., 1973). Dukor was able to show that in mice with a temporary inhibition of the complement system, a complete inhibition of the usual follicular localisation of the antigens was observed. He thus suggested that C3 has a pathogenetic role of particular importance in the control of the immunological response.

Recently Dukor tried to study some biochemical reactions – all complement-dependent – which may be responsible for the positive feed-back mechanism of the chronic inflammatory process:

1. The production of CSA (colony-stimulating activity) is responsible for the differentiation of macrophages and leukocytes from stem cells;

2. The production of neutral proteases and of plasminogen activator produces a further splitting of C3;

3. The production of lymphocyte-activating factor (LAF) enhances antibody synthesis and immune complexes formation;

4. Both immune complexes and C3b further activate the complement system via classic and alternative pathways;

5. The newly formed C3a activates other inflammatory cells from the circulation and induces the production of new mediators (Fig. 1).

On the basis of these experimental results it seems possible to broaden the field of interests related to the physiopathology of the serum complement system. The role played in acute inflammation is now well known and uniformly agreed, but the time is coming to evaluate the complement system in a new light, perhaps unexpected, but nevertheless very important, as modulator of the inflammatory response and of the possibility of transformation and self-maintenance of an acute process into a chronic one.

This last role, which should be typical of the C3 fraction, is still undefined but it is extremely important from a theoretical point of view, being one of the most interesting experimental proofs of the cooperation between humoral and cell-mediated immunity. It may then be argued that the serum complement

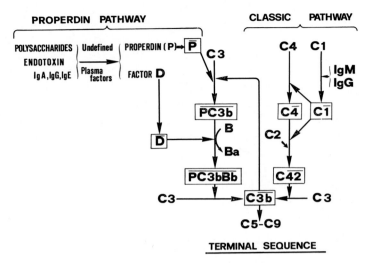

Fig. 1. Classic and alternative pathways of activation of the complement system (Fearon et al., 1973).

system is not only one of the main homeostatic mechanisms as modulator of the acute inflammation response, but also a possible linkage between T lymphocytes and B lymphocytes (which have long been considered independent of each other), thus giving a continuous integration of humoral and cell-mediated immune reactions (Fig. 2).

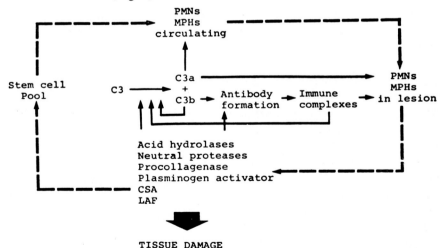

Fig. 2. Complement and the vicious circle of mediator release from inflammatory cells (Dukor et al., 1974).

Activation of complement system

In standard conditions, the serum complement system is inactive, but potentially active. Its activation, performed through a complex series of biological phenomena, is dependent on some modifications of the single components at the molecular level. These reactions are not yet completely understood. Activation follows a sequential mechanism, something like the activation of the other plasma protein systems such as coagulation, fibrinolysis and kinin synthesis. The enzymatic processes which are at the basis of the transformation of the single components from inactive to active status are self-controlled, in the sense that no one step can be achieved until the conclusion of the previous one. These enzymatic reactions are automatically controlled, being modulated, at different levels, by regulating processes dependent on the activating processes of other plasma protein systems, the production of particular substances by the inflammatory cells, and the interaction with the inhibitory substances, which have a specific action limited to only one level of activation.

As stated above, the different components of the serum complement system have been physico-chemically identified and isolated with different methods. From a functional point of view, the serum complement system should be divided into three parts: two possible pathways of activation are known, the classic and the properdin one, both causing C3 activation, from which the third phase starts, as represented by the activation from C3 to C9. This type of activation is 'sequential' and 'obliged'.

The classic pathway of activation starts with the transformation of C1 from inactive to active status. The active status of C1 has esterase-like properties. This transformation is usually induced by immune complexes or by aggregated IgG or IgM. The esterase activity of C1 activates C4 and C2 components. During this reaction a few fragments are obtained and one of these, known as C42 activated, is the C3 convertase, which then activates C3 and the rest of the sequence until C9 is reached (Table 1 and Fig. 2).

The molecular interactions of the properdin pathway are more complicated and not completely understood. Sometimes the primary induction of this type of activation may be to due to polysaccharides, both endotoxins and not, and to immunoglobulins (IgA and IgM but not IgG). These activating substances probably interact with properdin, a proesterase known as D factor, and with other unknown factors. The result is the activation of both properdin and D factor. This last factor seems to be the convertase of C3 proactivator. The activated properdin, and perhaps even the activated D factor, should act overall on C3; the product of this interaction is PC3b fragment, which should induce the activation of C3 proactivator by the activated D fragment and the consequent production of at least two other fragments, one minor, C3a, and one major, Bb. The final substance is probably a complex product called PC3Bb. This substance is the C3 convertase of the properdin pathway of complement activation and is functionally similar to the activated C42 complex of the classic line of complement activation, both being able to activate the system from C3 to C9 (Fearon et al., 1973).

The properdin should have a particular affinity for the C3d fragment. These two factors joined together act on C3bBb convertase, increase its half-life in vitro and enhance the further activation process. The C3b activated fragment, which is a result of the proteolytic action of the two convertases on C3, enhances the properdin pathway of activation by a feed-back mechanism: in this way a process of amplification of the activation of the last unit, and a monodirectional 'necessary' linkage between the classic and properdin pathways of activation should be possible. This last pathway of complement activation might be stimulated a second time by the production of activated C3b, even if the convertase is the C42 activated factor, i.e. the specific one of the classic line of complement activation (Fig. 1 and Table 1).

TABLE 1

Differences between the classic and alternative pathway of activation of the complement system

| | Pathway | |
	Classic	Alternate
Activating Ig	IgG, IgM	IgG, IgA, IgE
Activation site	Fc	F(ab')2 Fc
Participation of C1, C4 and C2	essential	none
Divalent cation requirements	$Ca^{++}Mg^{++}$	Mg^{++}
C3 cleaving enzyme	C3 convertase (C42)	C3 activator

This brief review of the serum complement system may be useful to evaluate the key role of C3 factor, which joins the two pathways of activation along the classic and properdin lines. In both cases the whole activity of the system, studied for instance by immune hemolysis, is lowered as a consequence of the utilisation of the last components. In both cases a proportional lowering of C3 concentration should be found, but if the activation of the serum complement is made along the classic pathway, there will be a proportional lowering of the first components C1, C4 and C2. In contrast, if activation follows the properdin pathway, the concentration of these three components will be normal, while the specific components of the properdin line (such as properdin, C3 proactivator, C3 activator and, of course, C3) will be reduced.

All these data have an inherent biological significance, because they allow a better understanding of the functional activity of the serum complement system, and are of clinical interest. In fact, even if the evaluation of the whole complement activity and of the concentration of the single components in biological fluids has a static significance, being the picture of a previous clinical phenomenon, these types of clinical tests, especially if repeated and correlated with immunohistochemical studies, still appear very interesting and stimulating, and suggest a possible new role for the serum complement system in the broad spectrum of host-reactive changes.

Activation of the complement system and acute inflammation

As we have previously underlined, the sequential reactivity of the serum complement system is one of the main features of acute inflammation. There are two particularly important aspects of this participation: one is linked to the multi-molecular aggregate which is adherent to the target cells, which may be a bacterium and which will produce the cytolysis; and the other is linked to the release into the body's fluids of substances known as chemical mediators of inflammation. These mediators have been studied for a long time, to the point that pharmacological research led to the production of a series of specific inhibitors of one or more chemical mediators, for a better understanding of the pharmacological basis of inflammation.

It now seems that the production of chemical mediators of acute inflammation is a relatively late phenomenon, when the activation of plasma systems has already occurred. However, at this stage the inflammatory cells have not yet started to participate in the process. In other words, it seems possible that the activation of plasma protein systems comes before, and perhaps modulates, the synthesis and release of the chief chemical mediators.

We are thus justified in considering the dynamics of acute inflammation as a series of consecutive phases, following Willoughby and Di Rosa (1971). The first phase seems to be represented by the primary cellular lesion which triggers off the next phases; the second is characterised by the activation of plasma protein systems; the third by the production of the chemical mediators, and the fourth by the activation of inflammatory cells.

The production of chemical mediators is thus an advanced stage of the inflammatory process, which follows the activation of the proteic systems. Among these, the serum complement system appears to be one of the most important.

Two points may be helpful for a better understanding of the problem:

1. The production of chemical mediators follows a chronological schedule: if we look at edema from carrageenan in the rat leg as an experimental model, we see that the growing volume of the leg follows the release, first of all of histamine and serotonin, then of kinins, and later on of prostaglandins. If the animals are treated with specific inhibitors, it may be possible to block the histamine-serotonin phase, or the kinin phase, or the prostaglandin phase, depending on the type of inhibitor used (Willoughby et al., 1969). These inhibitors act on the mediator and not on the process of production.

2. If we block complement activation, for instance with a specific antiserum as reported by Willoughby, all three phases will be inhibited.

The experimental observations are consistent with a relationship between the mechanisms of production of chemical mediators and the activation of the complement system. In this way the chronological criteria of precedence of complement activation are confirmed and the important role of this system in the development of the inflammatory process is further emphasized.

In Figure 3 the sequential phases and the phenomena characteristic of inflammation are shown. Particular value is attached to: (1) the key role of the

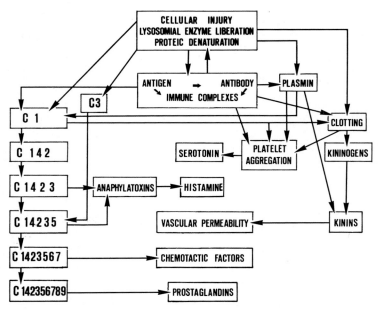

Fig. 3. Relationship between activation of the complement and production of chemical mediators. (From Willoughby and Di Rosa, 1971, modified.)

serum complement system in the different phases of inflammation; it should be stressed that the serum complement system participates in all types of inflammatory processes, not only in immune-mediated inflammation, as previously thought; (2) the relationship between the activation of the complement system and the other plasma systems; (3) the relationship between the different phases of activation of the complement system and the production of chemical mediators which – directly or indirectly – are all complement-dependent (Figs. 3 and 4).

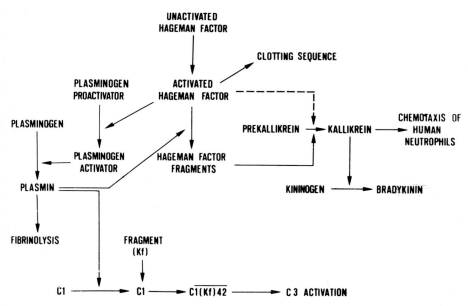

Fig. 4. Relationship between activation of the complement and activation of the other plasma protein systems. (Gigli and Nelson, 1968)

Relationships between complement activation and production of chemical mediators

As is well known to everyone in this field, the number of substances produced during the induction of acute inflammation is very high, and probably not yet completely known. From a chemical point of view, these mediators may be grouped as follows:

Proteases: plasmin, kallikrein, and the so-called globulinic factor of permeability.

Polypeptides: leukotaxine, kallidin, bradykinin.

Amines: histamine and serotonin.

Fat acids: prostaglandins.

Other substances: granulocytic substance; lymph node permeability substance (LNFF); slow reacting substance (SRS); colon contraction stimulating factor; platelet factor stimulating the hyperplasia of smooth muscle cells; cellular adherence factor.

This classification is certainly incomplete and not homogeneous, because for the identification of some mediators chemical criteria were followed, and for others functional criteria (when the molecular structure was unknown). As regards chemically defined mediators, their functional role appears especially in the so-called liquid phase of inflammation (i.e. not at the cellular level), acting on vascular permeability, vascular tone, chemotaxis of cellular elements, platelet aggregation and other phenomena related to the coagulation process. In more detail, it has been observed that the neutralisation of herpes simplex virus by a specific antiserum is not effective under some conditions, e.g. in the absence of C1 and C4. If the concentrations of these two components of the complement system are not high enough, the degree of neutralisation of the virus may be enhanced by the presence of C2 and C3 fractions. These are stages in the complicated mechanism of phagocytosis which seem to require the participation of more components of the serum complement system.

The phenomenon of immune adherence may be considered as a functional or integrated stage of the phagocytic process. Immune adherence is also complement-dependent: many cells have specific receptors for C3b fragment. These include red blood cells, leukocytes and platelets. Immune adherence enhances phagocytosis by polymorphonucleated leukocytes, with consequent release of lysosomal enzymes which may split the factors on C5 with production of C5a, membrane disruption and possible activation of Hageman factor (Gigli and Nelson, 1968).

A vasoactive substance has been isolated in patients affected by hereditary angioedema. This substance is different from bradykinin (Donaldson et al., 1969) and could be a product of the splitting of C2 (Lepow, 1971). The activation of C3 produces C3a, which causes degranulation of peritoneal mast cells in rats, contraction of the isolated ileum of guinea pigs and a hyperemic and hyperthermic edema when injected subcutaneously in man (Lepow, 1971).

All these properties characterize an anaphylotoxic substance which is also found as a product of the splitting of C5, i.e. C5a, which shows chemotactic activity for polymorphonucleated leukocytes and monocytes (Ward et al., 1965, 1971). A similar chemotactic activity has been attributed to the trimolecular complex C5C6C7. It has been thought that C6 participates even in blood clotting processes (Zimmerman and Muller Eberhard, 1971), acting on the biological functions of platelets. It has been demonstrated that the platelet-mediated allergic response related to the activation of C3 cannot be evoked in rabbits with a C6 deficiency. All these data tend to confirm that C6 is of fundamental importance in the allergic lysis of platelets. In addition, it has been shown that the whole coagulation process is defective in rabbits with a C3 deficiency, and that this phenomenon should be related to faulty platelet lysis, and release of platelet constituents.

We were able to demonstrate that platelet aggregation induced in vitro by ADP, norepinephrine or collagen consumes C3 and appears to be highly modified by previous activation with zymosan, inulin or endotoxin along the alternative pathway (Figs. 5–10). We think that all these data, even if necessarily incomplete, clearly show the need for a deeper study of the role of complement in the acute inflammatory process.

Relationship between activation of complement system and activation of other plasma systems (coagulation, fibrinolysis, kinins)

It is widely accepted that bradykinin synthesis in human blood is dependent on the activation of Hageman factor by a series of biological substances (Ratnoff and Naff, 1967). Hageman factor induces the coagulation reaction, but in the meantime reacts with one or more plasma cofactors, such as the pro-activator of plasminogen, to start the fibrinolytic process through the con-

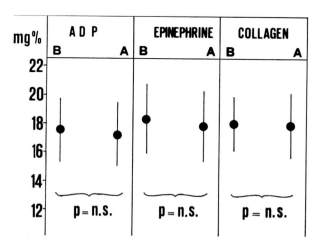

Fig. 5.   Concentration of Clq in PRP before and after platelet aggregation.

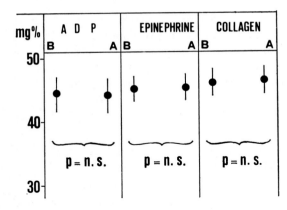

Fig. 6. Concentration of C4 in PRP before and after platelet aggregation.

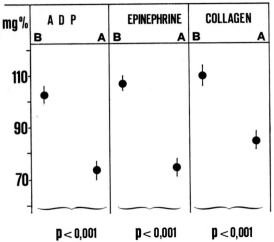

Fig. 7. Concentration of C3 (Beta 1C globulin) in PRP before and after platelet aggregation.

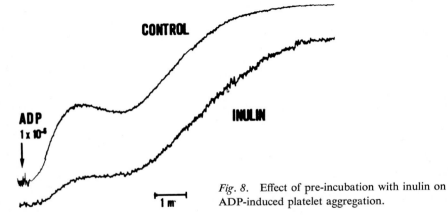

Fig. 8. Effect of pre-incubation with inulin on ADP-induced platelet aggregation.

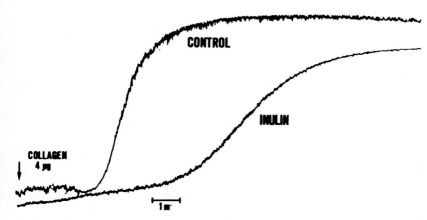

Fig. 9. Effect of pre-incubation with inulin on collagen-induced platelet aggregation.

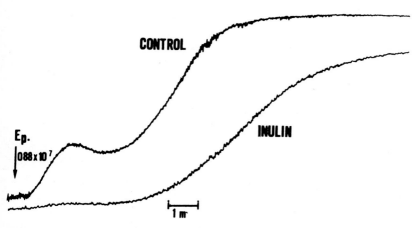

Fig. 10. Effect of pre-incubation with inulin on epinephrine-induced platelet aggregation.

version of plasminogen to plasmin (Ogston and Ratnoff, 1969). Plasmin seems to act through an enzymatic system on the activated Hageman factor with consequent synthesis of fragments which are able to activate the transformation of prekallikrein into kallikrein (Kaplan and Austen, 1970). The activation of the kallikrein system should be responsible for the transformation of kinin into bradykinin. These complicated relationships are not easy to understand from a biological point of view and more information is needed. We should put at the starting point of these reactions the Hageman factor, which induces the blood clotting process through the conversion of plasma precursors of thromboplastin into their activated form, interacting with one or more cofactors. The activation of the same Hageman factor starts the fibrinolytic process through the transformation of plasminogen into plasmin and directly activates prekallikrein, thus producing the series of reactions which lead to kinins formation. To this series of direct relationships between the activation of Hageman factor and other biological processes, we should add the indirect or second degree reactions. Plasmin, in fact, has an inherent proteolytic activity, such as transformation of fibrinogen and fibrin (fibrinolysis), C3 splitting with production of anaphylatoxin (Taylor and Ward, 1967) and activation of C1 (Ratnoff and Naff, 1967), which is followed by complement activation. In addition, kinin synthesis is followed by the production of a fragment (Kf) which activates C1, enhancing its reactivity with C4 and C2 and the production of C3 convertase.

In contrast, we have previously seen that the activation of the serum complement system, particularly the C3 component, is related to the process of platelet aggregation, thus acting also in the coagulation sequence. All these data, valuable from an analytical point of view, suggest a unitary interpretation of the inflammatory process such as that proposed by Willoughby and Di Rosa (1971).

Pharmacology of the complement system

In the last few years it has been postulated that it may be possible to interfere with the functions of the complement system with pharmacological agents. First an attempt was made to neutralize the chemical mediators, so anti-histaminic and anti-bradykininic agents, and other drugs active on vascular permeability, chemotaxis and platelet aggregation were isolated. Other research programs evaluated the possibility of isolating pharmacological agents able to block the activation of the complement system at different levels, following both the classic and alternative pathways of activation.

In previous papers we discussed the basic problems involved and the results of some experiments (Di Perri and Auteri, 1971, 1973, 1974a, b). In this paper we report a further improvement in the method previously used, particularly in order to control graphically the hemolytic reaction obtained using a turbidimeter and continuous registration system, and the selective reactivation of the complement system using purified human complement fraction. This study allowed us to understand a particular aspect of complement pharmacology which we think can be particularly useful to evaluate the properties of any new anti-inflammatory agent.

Material and methods

In all the studies concerning a prospective action on the activation of the complement system along the classic pathway, the serum complement activity has been expressed as 50% hemolytic units (CH_{50}). In addition the anticomplement activity and the identification of the site of action of the pharmacological agent were studied following the technique reported elsewhere (Di Perri and Auteri, 1971, 1973, 1974a, b). Only human serum complement was used (Figs. 11–14). On the other hand, in all the studies concerning a prospective action of the pharmacologic agent along the properdin pathway of activation of the complement system, we used a technique also based on hemolysis, but excluding any immunological interaction, i.e. hemolytic antibodies.

The hemolytic reaction is produced in a system characterized by sheep red blood cells, complement (fresh serum) and a polysaccharide, which in our system is represented by inulin. The amount of hemolysis which develops in this system is directly proportional to the potential activity of the properdin system following specific stimulation. The pharmacological agent is added in increasing concentrations without any pH change. If the pharmocological agent is able to inhibit hemolysis, the next step is to study the lowest quantity required for the total inhibition of the hemolytic process (Fig. 15).

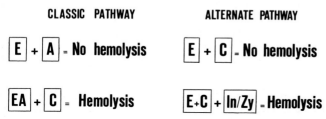

Fig. 11. Hemolysis along the classic and alternative pathway of activation of complement. E = erythrocytes, C = complement (fresh serum), A = hemolytic antibody, In = inulin, Zy = zymosan.

1st phase

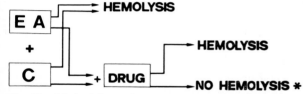

Fig. 12. Methodology of study of the anticomplementary activity of a pharmacologic agent (first phase). * = drug inhibits immune hemolysis.

2nd phase
NO HEMOLYSIS
HEMOLYSIS *
EA + C + DRUG
+ EA
NO HEMOLYSIS **
HEMOLYSIS **
+ C
NO HEMOLYSIS *

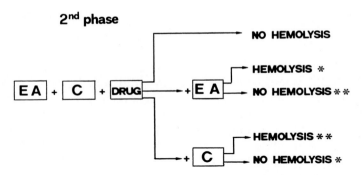

Fig. 13. Methodology of study of the anticomplementary activity of a pharmacologic agent (second phase). * = drug is active on EA; ** = drug is active on C.

3rd phase
EA+C+DRUG
+ C-C1
+ C-C4
+ C-C2
+ C-C3
HEMOLYSIS *
NO HEMOLYSIS **

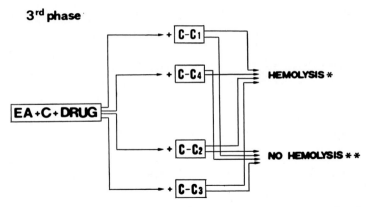

Fig. 14. Methodology of study of the anticomplementary activity of a pharmacologic agent (third phase). * = drug is not active on the missing component. ** = drug is active on the missing component.

E + C = no hemolysis
E C + Inulin = hemolysis
ALTERNATE PATHWAY
EC + Drug + Inulin
hemolysis
no hemolysis *

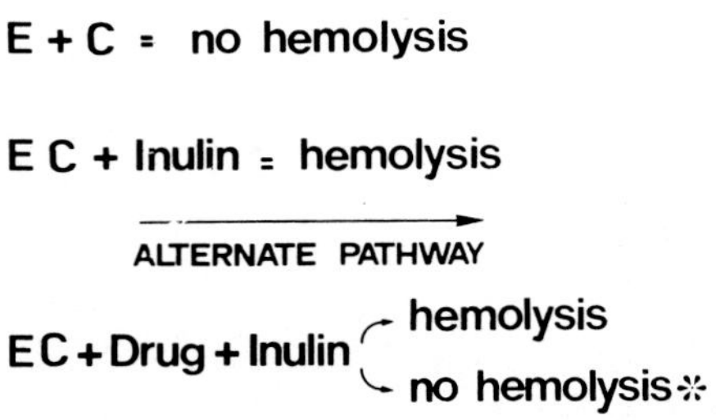

Fig. 15. Methodology of study of the anticomplementary activity of a pharmacologic agent (alternative pathway). * = drug inhibits the alternative pathway of complement activation.

Experiments on dynamics

The studies we performed following the technique described, particularly those related to the pharmacology of the serum complement system and the identification of the pharmacological agents able to interfere with the activation process, evaluated the grade of hemolysis (both immunologically and not non-immunologically mediated) with a spectrophotometric investigation made at a specific wave length. In this way we obtained a static evaluation of the phenomenon, having only the final result of all the reactions. For this reason, we tried to follow the dynamics of the hemolysis, both immunologically and non-immunologically mediated. This was possible by utilising an original method of continuous recording in experimental conditions which were differently modulated.

To study the dynamics of the hemolytic process we used a turbidimeter consisting of a source of continuous light, a filter with a wave length of 609 nm, and a little cuvette with a prefixed temperature of 37°C which was interposed between the light source and the photoelectric cell, and, following the change of transparency of the cuvette, sent signals which were recorded by a calibrated writing recorder. The strength of the signal was calculated on the scale 0–100, which represent 0% and 100% transmission respectively. The composition at 0 is as follows:

hemolysis following the classic pathway (EA system)

    0.5 ml of sheep red blood cells at 3% concentration (1.5×10^5),

    0.5 ml of hemolytic antibodies diluted at 1/800 (titre not less than 5000),

    1.5 ml of normal saline.

hemolysis following the alternative pathway (E system)

    1 ml of sheep red blood cells at 5% concentration (2.5×10^5),

    1.5 ml of normal saline.

100 transmission means total hemolysis, which is obtained in the two different systems described above with the addition of 1.5 ml of distilled water, instead of normal saline. With this apparatus it is possible to draw a graph with the transmission changes on the ordinate and the time in minutes on the abscissa.

For the study of the dynamics of the classic pathways of complement activation, the composition of the hemolytic system is as follows: 0.5 ml sheep red blood cells at 3% concentration; 0.5 ml hemolytic antibodies (titre not 5,000) diluted at 1/800. When recording starts we add 1.5 ml of fresh human serum diluted at 1/50 to the system previously prepared in the little cuvette. We prefer to use barbital buffer enriched with Ca^{++} and Mg^{++} at pH 7.4 as the diluting solution.

For the study of the dynamics of the alternative pathway of activation of complement, the composition of the hemolytic system is: 1 ml sheep red blood cells at 5% concentration; 1.5 ml fresh human serum diluted at 1/50. When recording starts we add 100 μl zymosan (suspension in barbital buffer 4 mg/ml) or 40 μl inulin (suspension in barbital buffer 10 mg/ml) to the system previously prepared in the cuvette.

Recording was followed for between 10 and 30 minutes until the phenomenon was not sufficiently clearly completed.

In these first experiments on the dynamics of complement activation, we examined the following problems which were previously studied by traditional methods: (1) complement depletion by zymosan and hemolytic reaction along the classic pathway; (2) relationship between incubation time with zymosan and hemolytic reaction along the alternative pathway; (3) inhibition of immunological hemolysis (classic pathway) and reactivation of the system by fresh serum and purified fractions of human complement.

As far as the first problem was concerned, all experiments were performed as described above, using the immune hemolytic standard system as control. In fact, the serum added to the EA system to have the first standard line is incubated also with a prefixed dose of zymosan for 30, 60 and 120 minutes at 37°C. (Figs. 16, 17). The next three lines are the graphic recording of the hemolysis mediated by sera and incubated with the EA system following the technique previously described.

As regards the second problem, all the experiments were performed as described, following the non-immune hemolysis (E system). As control line,

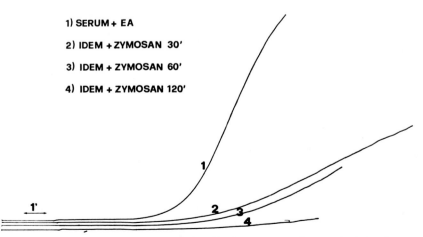

1) SERUM + EA

2) IDEM + ZYMOSAN 30'

3) IDEM + ZYMOSAN 60'

4) IDEM + ZYMOSAN 120'

Fig. 16. Dynamics of hemolysis: relationship between complement depletion by zymosan and hemolytic reaction along the classic pathway.

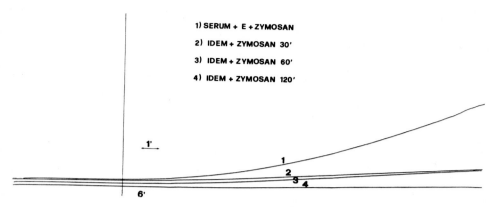

1) SERUM + E + ZYMOSAN

2) IDEM + ZYMOSAN 30'

3) IDEM + ZYMOSAN 60'

4) IDEM + ZYMOSAN 120'

Fig. 17. Dynamics of hemolysis: relationship between time of incubation by zymosan and hemolytic reaction along the alternative pathway.

that obtained by adding zymosan at 0 time was used, i.e. serum, sheep red blood cells and zymosan placed simultaneously in the cuvette. The next lines of hemolysis were obtained by adding to the serum (previously incubated for 30, 60 and 120 minutes with zymosan) the sheep red blood cells.

As regards the third problem, the experiments were performed as above, following the immune hemolytic standard system. The next lines may be divided into two different phases, the first being the graphic record of hemolysis inhibition with a fixed dose of indometacin, the second representing the attempt to reconstitute the complement activity by adding fresh serum or purified fractions of human complement (C1, C2, C3, C4).

Results and conclusions

As regards the study of the pharmacological activity of some agents on the complement system performed following the method described elsewhere, the results were reported in previous papers (Di Perri and Auteri, 1971, 1973, 1974a, b). We tried to complete our experiments with the second experimental model (previously described), i.e. the alternative pathway using inulin as activator. From Table 2 it appears that inhibition of the activation of the properdin pathway, i.e. absence of hemolysis, may be obtained only with some pharmacologic agents. All these drugs act not only on the activation of the complement along the classic pathway, but also at the level of the third component, as we previously showed in our original screening system.

TABLE 2

Action of some drugs on complement activation

Classic pathway Affected component		Alternate pathway
1.	Acetylsalicylic acid 9 × 10⁻⁴ M	— — — —
2. 4. 3.	Indometacin 2 × 10⁻³ M	+ + +
4. 3.	Phenylbutazone 3 × 10⁻³ M	+ + +
3.	Mefenamic acid 1.2 × 10⁻⁴ M	+ + +
3.	Flufenamic acid 1.6 × 10⁻⁴ M	+ + +
3.	Heparin	+ + +
4.	Cinnarizine 7 × 10⁻⁵ M	+ + +
4.	Cinnarizine 7 × 10⁻⁵ M + 0.1 ml 0.1 M MgCl₂	— — — —
3.	Clofibrinic acid	+ + +
1. 4.	DA 2370 (zepelin)	— — — —
1. 4.	Dipyridamole	— — — —
1. 4.	Frusemide	— — — —

The only exception is cinnarizine, which however has a proper pharmacologic activity as regards its anticomplementary action. As we have earlier reported, the action of this agent is magnesium-dependent, and it is well known that magnesium is absolutely necessary to activate the properdin pathway. The validity of our hypothesis concerning the magnesium-dependent activity of cinnarizine was confirmed by the reappearance of hemolysis on adding MgCl₂ to the hemolytic system.

The experiments on the dynamics of complement activation show the value of this new method for studying hemolysis.

Figure 16, showing the classic pathway of activation, shows what was partly known, i.e. that the line first has a latent phase, then a sudden rise and finally a plateau.

Figure 17 shows the activation along the properdin pathway and is completely different. First of all, there is a long period during which the red blood cells remained unchanged, then a gradual, slow and progressive hemolysis starts, following a relatively rectilinear course. It should be noted that all the experiments had a standard control for spontaneous hemolysis, so the phenomena appear to be related to the experimental conditions.

As regards the activity of zymosan on immune hemolysis, there is no doubt that the incubation period influences the highest grade of hemolysis and the speed of rise of the hemolysis curve (Fig. 16). All these data resemble those reported in the world literature on the possible depletion of C3 fraction by zymosan. Probably it is not a depletion of C3 as specific competition against the enzymatic process of activation, but rather a direct activation of the complement system beyond C3, thus giving a depletion of all the components (C3–C9) with an ensuing reduction of the strength of the hemolytic system. This hypothesis was confirmed by the results obtained by preincubating zymosan with the non-immune hemolytic system (which is stimulated along the alternative pathway).

If we add zymosan to the system, we obtain a certain degree of hemolysis, which is reduced and disappears when zymosan is incubated with the serum before adding the washed red blood cells.

In our last experiments on the dynamics of complement activation we documented the inhibition of immune hemolysis by indometacin (Fig. 18). The

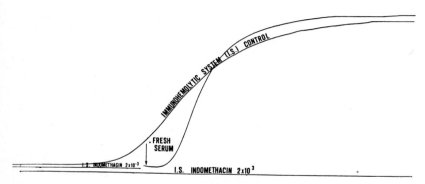

Fig. 18. Dynamics of hemolysis: graphic representation of the reactivation of the complement (blocked by indometacin) by a new dose of fresh serum.

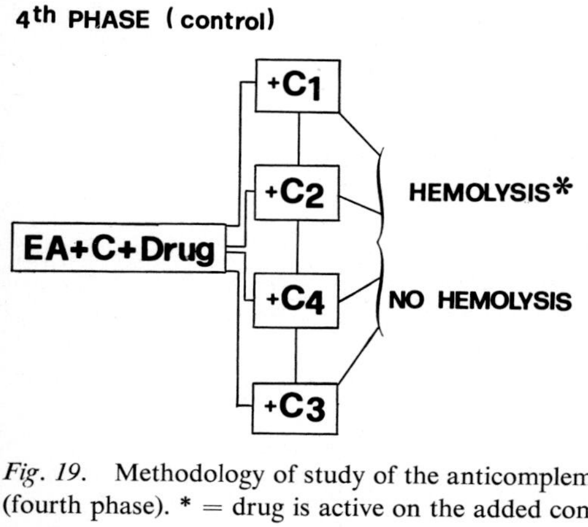

4th PHASE (control)

```
                    ┌──┤+C1│
                    │
                    │  ┌──┤+C2│     HEMOLYSIS *
   ┌────────────┐   │  │
   │ EA+C+Drug  ├───┤  │
   └────────────┘   │  │  ┌──┤+C4│  NO HEMOLYSIS
                    │
                    └──┤+C3│
```

Fig. 19. Methodology of study of the anticomplementary activity of a pharmacologic agent (fourth phase). * = drug is active on the added component(s).

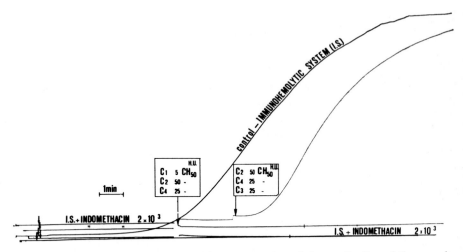

Fig. 20. Dynamics of hemolysis: graphic representation of the reactivation of the complement blocked by indometacin by purified fractions of human complement.

rise after the addition of a new dose of fresh serum confirm our previous results with the spectrophotometric model. In addition, we were able to confirm the validity of our screening system using purified human complement fractions. The site of indometacin activity at the level of the second, third and fourth component of complement is confirmed by the reappearance of hemolysis after the addition of sufficient doses of human complement purified fractions (obtained from Cordis Co., Miami, U.S.A.) described above. Thus the graph of the phenomenon shows a sudden rise (Figs. 19 and 20).

All these data, even if still incomplete, suggest the possibility of studying some phenomena which may be useful from a biological and pharmacological point of view.

References

BIANCO, C., NUSSENZWEIG, V. and MAYER, M. M. (1973): C3 split products inhibit the binding of antigen-antibody complement complexes to B lymphocytes. *J. Immunol.*, *110*, 1452.

BOKISCH, V. A., MULLER EBERHARD, H. J. and COCHRANE, C. G. (1969): Isolation of a fragment (C3a) of the third component of human complement containing anaphylotoxin and chemotactic activity and description of an anaphylotoxin inactivator of human serum. *J. exp. Med.*, *129*, 1109.

DI PERRI, T. and AUTERI, A. (1971): Effect of some pyrimido-pyrimidinic compounds on the complement. In vitro and in vivo studies. First Meeting of European Division of International Society of Hematology. In: *Aggregazione Piastrinica*, p. 81. Boeringher, Ingelheim.

DI PERRI, T. and AUTERI, A. (1973): Anticomplementary properties of cinnarizine. *Arch. Int. Pharm. Ther.*, *203*, 23.

DI PERRI, T. and AUTERI, A. (1974a): On the anticomplementary action of some non-steroidal anti-inflammatory drugs. In: *Future Trends in Inflammation*, p. 215. Piccin Medical Books.

DI PERRI, T. and AUTERI, A. (1974b): Interesse di una ricerca sull'attività dei farmaci anti-flogistici sull'attivazione del sistema complementare. *Riv. Farmacol. Ter.*, *5*, 213.

DONALDSON, V. H., RATNOFF, O. D. and DIAS DA SILVA, W. (1969): Permeability increasing activity hereditary angioedema plasma. *J. clin. Invest.*, *48*, 642.

DUKOR, P. and HARTMAN, K. (1973): Bound C3 as the second signal for B cells activation. *Cell. Immunol.*, *7*, 385.

DUKOR, P., SCHUMANN, G., GISLER, F. J., DIERICH, M. and BITTER SUERMAN, P. (1974): Complement dependent B cells activation by cobra venon factor and other mitogens. *J. exp. Med.*, *139*, 337.

FELDMANN, M. and PEPYS, M. B. (1974): Role of C3 in lymphocyte cooperation in vitro. *Nature (Lond.)*, *259*, 159.

FEARON, D. T., AUSTEN, K. F. and RUDDY, S. J. (1973): Formation of a hemolytically active cellular intermediate by the interaction between properdin factor B and D and the activated third component of complement. *J. exp. Med.*, *138*, 1305.

GIGLI, I. and NELSON, R. A. (1968): Complement dependent immune phagocytosis. *Exp. Cell. Res.*, *51*, 45.

KAPLAN, A. P. and AUSTEN, K. F. (1970): A prealbumin activator of prekallikrein. *J. Immunol.*, *105*, 802.

LEPOW, I. H. (1971): Permeability producing peptide product of the interaction of the first, fourth and second component of complement. In: *Biochemistry of Acute Allergic Reaction: Second International Symposium*, p. 205. Editors: Austen and Becker. Blackwell, London.

OGSTON, D. and RATNOFF, O. D. (1969): Studies on a complex mechanism for the activation of plasminogen by kaolin and by chlorophorm: the participation of Hagemann factor and additional cofactors. *J. clin. Invest.*, *48*, 1786.

PEPYS, M. B. and BUTTERWORTH, A. E. (1974): Inhibition by C3 fragments of C3 dependent rosette formation and antigen induced lymphocyte transformation. *Clin. exp. Immunol.*, *18*, 273.

RATNOFF, O. D. (1969): Some relationship among hemostasis, fibrinolitic phenomena, immunity and the inflammatory response. *Advanc. Immunol.*, *10*, 145.

RATNOFF, O. D. and NAFF, G. B. (1967): The conversion of Cls to Cl esterase by plasmin and trypsin. *J. exp. Med.*, *125*, 337.

TAYLOR, F. B. and WARD, P. A. (1967): Generation of chemotactic factor in rabbit serum by plasminogen-streptokinase mixture. *J. exp. Med.*, *126*, 149.

WARD, P. A., COCHRANE, C. G. and MULLER EBERHARD, H. J. (1965): The role of serum complement in chemotaxis of leucocytes in vitro. *J. exp. Med.*, *122*, 327.

WARD, P. A., OFFEN, C. D. and MONTGOMERY, J. F. (1971): Chemoattractans of leucocytes with special reference in lymphocytes. *Fed. Proc.*, *30*, 1721.

WILLOUGHBY, D. A., COOTE, C. D. and TURK, J. L. (1967): Complement in acute inflammation. *J. Path.*, *97*, 295.

WILLOUGHBY, D. A. and DI ROSA, M. (1971): A unifying concept for inflammation: a new appraisal of some mediators. In: *Immunopathology of Inflammation*, p. 28. Editors: B. K. Forscher and J. C. Houk. Excerpta Medica, Amsterdam.

ZIMMERMAN, T. S. and MULLER EBERHARD, H. J. (1971): Blood coagulation initiation by a complement mediated pathway. *J. exp. Med.*, *134*, 1601.

II. *Evaluation of non-steroidal anti-inflammatory drugs*

Chairman   C. B. Ballabio
Co-chairman H. C. Burry

Introduction

C. B. Ballabio

Istituto di Reumatologia, University of Milan, Italy

Recently we have seen the introduction of a host of drugs, all of which are claimed to have quite important therapeutical properties in the most widely differing rheumatic diseases.

Apart from the fact that these diseases are so recalcitrant to treatment that prudence must be exercised in judging the effectiveness of any medication in rheumatological therapy, the very proliferation of drugs licensed on the market is a reason for being cautious and critical when evaluating their effectiveness. What is needed is an attitude of cautious reserve based on rigorous application of methods, as well as ethical and economic imperatives, the latter being particularly important in a time of economic regression such as we now have in all but a few countries of the world.

Getting down to detailed evaluations, I would like to begin with pre-clinical trials and express my opinion, which is shared by others, that the results of pharmacological tests are too easily transposed in clinical practice. Without indulging in too drastic statements (namely, that no experimental effect in animals may stand surety for the future results of clinical work), we are bound to admit that the pathogenesis of experimental arthritis, which is the standard pharmacological test, has nothing or very little in common with human pathology.

Nobody denies the importance of such tests in so far as they are intended to investigate the biological action, to quantitate dosage, and to have a preliminary trial on the toxicity of the substances to be used in man. But we do not think that such tests should serve as evidence of the effectiveness of a drug or of its potency, particularly as regards information given to the doctor, investigator and practitioner. I will come back to this point of the responsibility of laboratories, but first I would like to emphasize some basic points about the many difficulties encountered in clinical experimentation, from the point of view of an adequate approach to and accomplishment of trials in man.

One of the most important points involved is the selection of patients. For years now we have stressed the importance of distinguishing the patients to be submitted to trials into 'cooperative' and 'non-cooperative' subjects, the two groups being characterized by different psychological attitudes which may have a considerable effect on the results of the trials. This preliminary consideration has acquired paramount importance in recent times, since ethical and political considerations demand (and possibly rightly so) that the patient to be submitted to a trial should be properly informed. Prof. Thompson, the author of a brilliant report presented at the Congress held at Torremolinos in 1975, states in this connection:

'We will try and obtain the patient's consent, possibly in writing, after explaining to him the nature, the purpose and the risk of treatment, if any. We shall recognize the patient's right to refuse participation in the trial, without any prejudice against him because of a refusal. These moral imperatives stand as a guarantee for each and every patient.'

I admit I fully agree with this statement from a formal point of view, but then on a practical level this sort of behaviour would in my opinion raise unsurmountable difficulties for adequate experimental clinical work. It is easy to infer in effect that the preliminary informing of the patient will lead to selection in favour of 'cooperative' subjects, and therefore yield more favourable responses, in that 'non-cooperative' subjects are excluded from the trial.

Even when preliminary information is as precise as possible, it is easy to understand that the patient's attitude will vary depending on his culture, his mentality, education, emotionality. All of us have come to observe regional differences, for instance, in the evaluation of results.

Another most delicate point is related to trials on in-patients as opposed to those on out-patients. It is trite but extremely significant that the in-patient, by the very fact that he is almost completely at rest, will be susceptible to a marked or even remarkable spontaneous improvement. What would we recommend: should we nowadays fix the hospitalization period required before starting the trial? Would that period be tolerable in economic terms? Who should pay for it? To what extent does each of us respect, or rather can each of us respect, this indispensable preliminary consideration? Very seldom do I read in papers that the patient was on a regime of physical activity for a period of two weeks, to say the very least! From that point of view, it would be better to rely on out-patients, who do not change their way of living during the trial. However, they often elude rigorous control as far as the regular taking of the drug, the determination of results and the timely detection of side effects are concerned.

Out-patients, however, are indispensable for long-term studies, the most reliable ones for the therapeutic evaluation of a drug. How often is the value of a drug sharply reduced after a while; how often does the drug utterly fail to stand the test of time!

Another point in line with the previous considerations is the environment, i.e. the place of the trials. In my opinion, rigorous specialization is required for a correct identification of the nature and severity of the disease, and to create competent specialized teams to determine objective findings.

I have no hesitation in expressing my whole-hearted support for some findings of exhaustive statistical investigations intended to interpret the different results obtained by various investigators, as reported by Prof. Lucchelli at the recent Symposium held in Tyrrhenia.

The need for careful selection of trial cases is best satisfied in specialized surgeries or hospitals. This also because of the easy choice of the most suitable subjects, so that the dangers described above can be avoided. It is my considered opinion (and I fully agree with Prof. Thompson on this) that a pilot experiment developed as an 'open' trial on patients well-informed about the therapeutical value of the most widely differing drugs taken through the course of their disease (patients whose personality and rigorous judgement are well known to us) will give us very reliable information as to the real value of the new drug.

All such considerations culminate in the evaluation of results, where we are bound to recognize that standardized methods are far from being achieved. The International Society of Rheumatology was fully aware of the problem and set up an ad hoc committee of which I am honoured to be a member. The problem was so deeply felt that it gave rise to many of the congresses held recently, such as the present and the next symposia.

It is a pleasure for me to see so many Italian investigators in the audience, because this issue was very widely discussed and received great attention in Italy in recent times.

In this moment of frightful plight it is really a crushing responsibility to license the introduction of any drug whose real usefulness has not been clearly established, particularly with the availability of other far less expensive drugs of documented efficacy. Furthermore, we have to consider that the placebo effect may account for as much as 70% of cases and that a large part of our treatment is limited to a symptomatic effect.

I would like to make some recommendations to all drug-producing firms. First of all, as some laboratories are already doing, they should thoroughly inform their representatives with regard to the properties and indications of the drug under consideration. Owing to the great responsibility these people have in informing the practitioner, I would suggest that they be recruited from among specialists in the subject, or at least properly trained through courses, periodical lectures and refresher courses so that they are up to date with developments in rheumatological studies.

Last but not least, I would like to say a word to the people responsible for marketing, who are too prone to give general and extensive indications. The very term 'rheumatism' is as all-embracing as God's forgiveness, so that the term 'antirheumatic' appears most easily on the labels and brochures presenting the drug, often coupled with the term 'anti-inflammatory', as if the two expressions were interchangeable. Once again I would recommend that words should be added to notions, and not the other way round, even though the opposite attitude unfortunately prevails in the current way of thinking, to ward off the risk that any anti-inflammatory drug be regarded as a cure-all for rheumatic diseases.

Close collaboration between laboratories and investigators in experimental work should be uninterrupted and both should be present at all times in a trial, if only in order to specify the indications, doses (which may vary in time), limits of effectiveness and possible side effects.

Evaluation of non-steroidal anti-inflammatory drugs by means of experimental arthritis models

V. Pipitone and R. Numo

Istituto di Reumatologia, University of Bari, Italy

For reliable preclinical evaluation of a non-steroidal anti-inflammatory substance (NSAD), every investigation must be carried out in experimental models that resemble, to some extent, rheumatoid arthritis in man. This has led many authors to make various attempts to elaborate different models which might fulfil the criteria suggested by Kaplan (1966).

The arthritic syndrome must affect many joints, especially the distal joint, with a chronic involvement. This experimental arthritis has to fulfil the following criteria:

1. From the point of view of morbid anatomy, it has to show the presence of a proliferative synovitis, with a pannus, and erosive changes in the subchondral and hypertrophy with a villous character that is most marked near the joint cartilage;

2. From the point of view of histopathology the synovial membrane has to show cellular infiltration with a mononuclear cell pattern (lymphoid and plasma cell) and with an absence of polymorphonuclear cells which characterize septic experimental arthritis;

3. The experimental picture should have a chronic course and, if possible, be self-perpetuating.

Only a few experimental models can be reasonably assumed to meet enough of these criteria (according to the Kaplan hypothesis) to be a good working model; among these, there are, to some extent, the models carried out using immunological procedures.

The models used so far can be grouped as follows:

1. Experimental arthritis induced by microorganisms;
2. Experimental arthritis induced by bacterial products;
3. Experimental arthritis induced by endocrinological means;
4. Experimental arthritis provoked with immunological procedures;
5. Experimental arthritis induced by different techniques.

Experimental arthritis induced by microorganisms

These models are based on the hypothesis, supported by many authors, that rheumatoid arthritis might be due to an infectious agent. Among these models four experimental kinds of arthritis can be distinguished: (a) by bacteria; (b) by mycoplasma; (c) by bedsoniae; (d) by viruses.

Among the bacteria the most widely used agents are streptococci, *E. coli* and *Salmonella enteritidis*. By using *Streptococcus equisimilis* (Robert et al., 1968), an acute septic arthritis, highly destructive, not chronic, can be obtained. With the group A *Streptococcus haemolitans* (L form) Cook et al. (1969) obtained more encouraging results (as far as the aspect of chronicity is concerned); nevertheless, they were far from the picture of a model of a chronic arthritis. Similiar results were also reported by Martin et al. (1968), who injected intravenous *E. coli* in young rabbits; a picture of an acute septic arthritis developed.

An interesting inducible polyarthritis was first described by Volman and Collins (1973) in rats; using intravenously injected *Salmonella enteritidis*, a chronic arthritis developed (unlikely to be due to a septic-type mechanism), which strongly suggests the possible role of immunological phenomena. Moreover, in an experiment carried out by Mansson et al. (1968), guinea pigs were fed a protein-rich diet; a week later an abnormal bacterial pattern appeared with a high incidence of *Clostridium perfringens* and subsequently the animals showed disturbances of movement and swollen peripheral joints, along with increased ESR and hypergammaglobulinaemia. Joint deformities were observed after some months, while the joint lesions consisted of synovitis with a cell-rich exudate.

Good results have been obtained with Erysipelothrix (especially with the strain *rhusopathiae* in type *insidiosa*); the use of this strain resulted in a progressive arthritis (Sikes, 1968; Timoney and Berman, 1970) with changes of joint tissue (cartilage, synovium and bone), body weight loss and stiffness (Nohn and Utklev, 1970).

Following the initial outline of the hypothesis that mycoplasma may be involved in the aetiology of rheumatoid disease, a great amount of investigation has gone into attempts to experimentally induce rheumatoid-like arthritis. For this purpose various strains have been used: *M. arthritidis* (Cole et al., 1971), *M. gallisepticum* (Olson and Kerr, 1967), (Lamas da Silva and Adler, 1969), *M. mycoides* (Piercy, 1970), *M. pulmonis* (Barden and Tully, 1969) and *M. hyorhinis* (Ennis et al., 1972). The use of these strains in some experiments provoked the development of migratory polyarthritis with severe synovitis, strongly suggesting the histopathological pattern of human rheumatoid arthritis. None of these pictures were steady, and all showed a tendency to spontaneous regression; therefore the main feature of a long-standing, self-perpetuating and chronic lesion was absent.

M. pulmonis seems to be very active in C3H mouse (Taylor et al., 1974), in which it does induce the appearance of an arthritis after a period of 2–4 weeks (Harwick et al., 1973a). In some cases the lesion can be prolonged for a long time after the primary infection; this might possibly be related to an immunological mechanism (Sokoloff, 1973). Evidence supporting this hypothesis comes from the observation that the arthritic mice develop a delayed-type hypersensitivity reaction to synovial membrane antigens from normal inbred mice (Harwick et al., 1973b).

A more typical rheumatoid-like arthritis can be observed with some strains of Bedsoniae which induce a chronic arthropathy with a histological picture of synovial villi as well as lymphoid and mononuclear cell infiltration.

In connection with virus experimental arthritis, the models induced by psittacosis (Pierson, 1967), rubella (Ocra and Herd, 1971) and herpes simplex virus are worth mentioning. The inoculation of herpes simplex virus in the knee joint of rabbits results in a picture of chronic long-standing arthritis (Bacon et al., 1974) and, strikingly, in the involvement of the non-injected knee (Webb et al., 1973).

Experimental arthritis induced by bacterial products

Weissman et al. (1965) observed the development of a chronic arthritis in the knees of rabbits injected with streptolysin S. Subsequently, Taylor et al. (1972) demonstrated that arthritis can be related to the mitogenic fraction of streptolysin S, possibly acting by the stimulation of lymphocytes of the synovial membrane, which means that the arthritis could be due to a delayed-type immunological mechanism.

Various bacterial products have been used (the streptococci cell wall and the *Klebsiella pneumoniae* lipopolysaccharide fractions), but in no case has rheumatoid-like polyarthritis been obtained.

Experimental arthritis by endocrinological means

This type of arthritis is not worth dwelling on, because at the moment it cannot be used in the evaluation of anti-inflammatory substances. Most of the experiments were carried out in rats, using the following hormones: prolactin, STH, anterior pituitary extract and DOCA.

Experimental arthritis induced by immunological procedures

This type of arthritis is one of the most widely used models in rheumatology: on the other hand it has proved to be one of the most reliable means of evaluating the anti-inflammatory and immunosuppressive activity of a drug. Although it is experimentally possible to induce a model resembling human rheumatoid arthritis, many authors (Mowat and Garner, 1972) do not entirely agree that such experimental models can mimic completely the human pathology, since none of the experimental forms of arthritis sufficiently resemble the rheumatoid condition to suggest a closely related pathogenesis.

The first model was carried out by Pearson (1964), who was able to produce an adjuvant arthritis in rats. If rats are injected intradermally in the footpad with an oil in water emulsion containing dead tubercle bacilli (Freund's complete adjuvant), they develop a disease which has many parallels with Reiter's syndrome, Behçet's disease and Stevens-Johnson syndrome as well as rheumatoid arthritis. In addition polyarthritis with mononuclear infiltration and typical pannus formation, and skin lesions are seen at other sites of frequent stimulus (i.e. eyes, ears, skin etc.). However, not all strains of rats are able to develop this arthritis: it appears in 100% of Lewis rats, but the incidence is significantly lower in AVN rats (3%) (Zidek and Perlik, 1971). In Wistar AF/Han EMD SPF rats, the injection of Freund's adjuvant does not induce polyarthritis, but a chronic osteomyelitis (Mohr et al., 1974). Two weeks after the injection a polyarthritis of the small peripheral joints develops; it is characterized by long-standing activity and severe involvement of different organs (with uveitis, nephritis). The histological picture is very peculiar and shows many striking points of resemblance with that of rheumatoid arthritis (synovitis with villi and diffuse infiltration of lymphoid and mononuclear cells).

The pathogenesis of adjuvant arthritis has long been discussed; the most widely accepted hypothesis is that it may well result from delayed hyper-sensitivity to an antigenic component of mycobacterial wax (Jasin et al., 1973). Moreover, much evidence supports this hypothesis (Whitehouse et al., 1971): (1) arthritis can be suppressed by anti-lymphocyte serum; (2) arthritis can be passively transferred only by lymph node lymphoid cells; (3) arthritis dramati-cally improves with the drainage of lymphocytes of the thoracic duct; (4) penicillamine alleviates the course of polyarthritis in rats. (Baumgartner et al., 1974).

Pearson's model has subsequently been changed in order to obtain poly-arthritis that resembles, as much as possible, certain examples of human arthritis. The way of action of adjuvant can be enhanced and increased by carrageenan or by digitonin (Mizushima et al., 1970) or by the addition of ovalbumin (Davis, 1971; Consden et al., 1971; Belovic and Kinsella, 1973). Using this last model (adjuvant plus ovalbumin), it is possible to detect the presence of antigen-antibody complexes that play a basic role in the patho-genesis of the onset of the lesion inducing arthritis (Belovic and Kinsella,1973). The above-mentioned immune complexes are probably responsible, in a sub-sequent stage, for remarkable changes in the synovium as well as in cartilage by means of a typical vasculitis (Steinberg et al., 1973). Recently, a new ar-thritis experimental model carried out by using Freund's adjuvant plus colla-gen-soluble antigen has been introduced by Steffen and Wick (1971).

Undoubtedly, the most elegant and classic immunological method for pro-voking experimental arthritis to date is that introduced by Dumonde and Glynn (1962). They have shown that an arthritis virtually indistinguishable from rheumatoid arthritis can be induced in rabbits by the intra-articular injection of homologous or heterologous fibrin if the animals have been pre-viously made sensitive by intradermal injections of fibrin in Freund's complete adjuvant. This scheme has been used in the following experiments carried out in different animals by our group: (a) in *Macaca rhesus*, according to the tech-nique of Lucherini (Lucherini et al., 1965; Malaguzzi Valeri et al., 1971, 1972); (b) in rabbit, using the classic model of Dumonde and Glynn (Malaguzzi Valeri and Pipitone, 1972; Carrozzo et al., 1972; Numo et al., 1972); (c) again in rabbit, previously made silicotic by silica endotracheal spray, in which fibrin plus Freund complete adjuvant arthritis was induced; (d) other immu-nological methods.

Arthritis in M. rhesus

This model was used by our group in parallel experiments with Malaguzzi Valeri et al. (1971, 1972) and proved extremely interesting both from the clinical and histopathological point of view as well as for immunological results

Three weeks after sensitization with fibrin and Freund's complete adjuvant, the animals were intradermally injected with fibrin only, as a triggering injection. Subsequent injections of fibrin were made on the 360th and the 390th day, and a two-year follow-up observation was made. The arthritis obtained was typical and severe with dramatic impairment of joint function associated with an interesting finding in the joints: the wrists were swollen, mostly symmetrically, while the distal small joints presented red swelling of varying sizes and different degrees of pain. The polyarthritis had been long-standing (over a period of not less than 12 months); each later injection resulted in a clear flare-up of general and joint conditions, sometimes more severe than at the onset of the disease.

The histological features observed in the joint and periarticular lesions are worth describing: they included villous hypertrophy of the synovial membrane with proliferation of lining synovial cells, and beneath that fibroblastic proliferation with infiltration of mononuclear and lymphoid cells which took on the appearance of 'perivascular islands'; in some animals endarteritis pictures were taken.

Investigative observations. Following the initial outline of the immunological background of the disease obtained, many immunological parameters were monitored. Anti-human gammaglobulin antibodies were present during the sensitization phase at a mean average level of 1 : 40. No significant change was noted during the experiment, except at the last control, 2 years after the onset of the arthritis, when a remarkable decrease in these antibodies was found. In contrast, anti-rabbit gammaglobulin antibodies were absent during the latency phase, but appeared with a progressive increase up to the sixth month of joint disease on the onset of the arthritis. No remarkable behaviour of anti-horse or anti-macaca gammaglobulin antibodies was observed.

The results obtained from the macaca lymphocyte cultures with homologous synovial membrane antigen should be mentioned: when challenged with the related antigen the lymphocytes proved responsive (this was probably due to a delayed hypersensitivity immunity phenomenon). The lymphocyte responsiveness to the antigen lasted throughout the period of induction of arthritis, even when the progressive decrease in antibody level was occurring.

Arthritis in the NZW rabbit

The second model was the classic one of Dumonde and Glynn, using sensitization with heterologous fibrin plus Freund's complete adjuvant. The intra-articular triggering injection with only fibrin resulted in a typical monoarthritis.

The arthritis developed a month after the triggering injection, and was so severe that it crippled the animal; the joint appeared swollen for the effusion and the proliferation of synovial membrane as well, as could be well seen when the articular cavity was opened. From the onset the articular cartilage showed gross changes of the surface which were hyperaemic with more or less small chinks which sometimes ended with the involvement of cartilage matrix pattern and with the erosion of subchondral bone. The synovial membrane had a villous appearance with inflammatory infiltration of mononuclear (chiefly lymphocytic) cells; in some areas the clustering of these elements around acid mucopolysaccharide deposits could be seen.

As far as it was possible to investigate, no remarkable finding was obtained concerning the problem of humoral antibodies. Antigammaglobulin antibodies were undetectable both at the appearance of arthritis and over the whole duration of joint disease. The increased uptake of ^{3}H-labelled thymidine by lymphocytes from arthritic rabbits in culture with synovial membrane antigen might lead to the conclusion that delayed hypersensitivity does play a paramount role in the mechanism of adjuvant arthritis in the NZW rabbit.

One group of arthritic rabbits was treated with indometacin (Merck, Sharp and Dohme) (5 mg/kg as sodium salt by parenteral injection). The treatment was started on the same day on which the sensitization was performed. Our data suggest that indometacin was unable to prevent the appearance of arthritis, but had an anti-inflammatory effect, as shown by the findings of less severe involvement of general conditions and a lower degree of changes in the synovial membrane and articular cartilage of the rabbits to which the drug was given.

Adjuvant and fibrin arthritis with associated experimental silicosis

The third model was used in an attempt to reproduce in NZW rabbits a picture resembling Caplan's syndrome in man. Arthritis was induced according to the usual model of Dumonde and Glynn, while the silicosis was previously induced by means of a quartz powder (matches were between 1 and 3 μm). The animals were divided into 4 groups: (a) control; (b) silicotic; (c) arthritic; (d) silico-arthritic.

The joint involvement was more marked in the silico-arthritic group than in the arthritic one: the number of affected joints was higher, and the degree of changes was more severe. Furthermore, using the classic model of Dumonde and Glynn, a monoarthritis in the joint injected with the triggering dose can be obtained, while the development of a polyarthritis was noted in the silico-arthritic group. In fact joint involvement was present not only in the injected knee but also in the opposite one, and in other joints as well. In the most typical cases the articular capsule showed oedema, while the articular cartilage appeared seriously damaged due to the presence of regressive alterations of varying extent (Fig. 1).

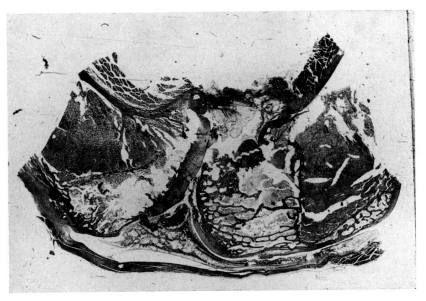

Fig. 1.   Silico-arthritic rabbits: articular cartilage shows regressive alterations.

In rabbits with silicosis plus arthritis the lesions were apparently more marked, while the processes appeared clearly phlogistic-haemorrhagic. The proliferation in the synovial membrane gave it a villous appearance, while in the articular cartilage the destroyed area appeared to be covered by fibrin-haemorrhagic material. The changes in the lungs of silicotic and silico-arthritic rabbits were investigated. In both groups granulomata with macrophages and lymphocytes and plasma cells were observed (Fig. 2); in addition, in the silico-arthritic group the presence of vasculitis with thickening of tunica media and infiltration and necrosis of the adventitious membrane was noted (Fig. 3).

The results of immunological screening were impressive: they included the detection of antirabbit (Waaler-Rose test) and antihuman (Ra test) gammaglobulin antibodies, and the lymphocyte transformation test. The Waaler-Rose test showed different behaviour in the 4 groups: the mean average was 1 : 16 in silicotic, between 1 : 16 and 1 : 32 in arthritic, and between 1 : 64 and

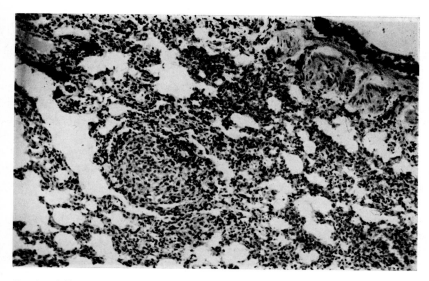

Fig. 2. Adjuvant and fibrin arthritis with associated experimental silicosis: granulomata with macrophages, lymphocytes, and plasma cells.

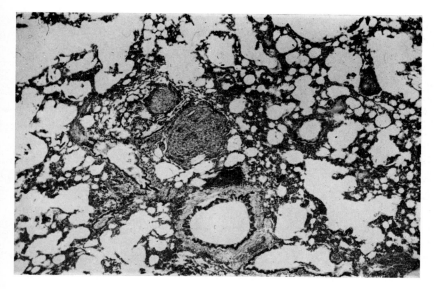

Fig. 3. Silico-arthritic rabbits: showing vasculitis with thickening of tunica media and infiltration and necrosis of the adventitious membrane.

1 : 128 (up to 1 : 256 in 1 case) in the silico-arthritic rabbits. The data on anti-human gammaglobulin antibodies was similar: in silicotic rabbits the mean average level was 1 : 80, in the arthritic ones between 1 : 80 and 1 : 320. and in the silico-arthritic ones between 1 : 160 and 1 : 320 (up to 1 : 640 in 1 case).

More difficult to interpret were the findings related to delayed hypersensitivity: the lymphocyte transformation test response with synovial membrane antigen, when calculated as blastic index, appeared higher in the lymphocyte population from arthritic rabbits than in silico-arthritic ones. On the other hand, when lung antigen was used, the blastic index was higher in lymphocyte cultures from silico-arthritic rabbits than in arthritic ones.

The results gained from the use of these three models leads to the conclusion that the immunological mechanism, on which they are based, can be considered to be one of the most effective in experimental rheumatology, since it does cause an arthropathy in many respects resembling the picture of human rheumatoid arthritis. This view is reasonably supported by clinical, histopathological, gross anatomical findings, and long duration as well. Related to this is the observation of Glynn (1975) in rabbits with experimental arthritis, in which 2–3 years after the onset of the disease, the joint presented the signs of an inflammatory process. On the basis of these results, it may be claimed that the model of Dumonde and Glynn – in the original technique, as well as in the modification we introduced – provides a highly reliable model for the evaluation of the activity and mechanism of anti-inflammatory drugs which are continuously introduced in rheumatology.

Other immunological methods

Brouilhet et al. (1975) introduced an experimental model very similar to that of Dumonde and Glynn: ovalbumin was used as antigen, while the adjuvant in some cases contained *M. tuberculosis* and in others *M. butyricum*. In the early stages the arthritis which appeared was similar for both the adjuvants, but in subsequent stages arthritis persisted only in the animals in which *M. tuberculosis* adjuvant was injected. This led the authors to the conclusion that self-perpetuation is strictly linked to the action of *M. tuberculosis*, which is more powerful than *M. butyricum* as adjuvant. Ovalbumin only serves to initiate the inflammatory process.

The role of delayed hypersensitivity in the pathogenesis of rheumatoid arthritis has long been discussed. In order to give support to this hypothesis many authors performed a series of experiments injecting different mediators of delayed hypersensitivity into the knees of rabbits (MIF, blastogenic factor, etc.). Andreis et al. (1975) were thus able to produce a chronic inflammatory process. Other immunological models are quite different from the classic one of Dumonde and Glynn; of these it is worth mentioning the one used by Rawson et al. (1969), who produced a picture of chronic synovitis by injecting the Fab fragment of immunoglobulins into the joints of rabbits.

In some experiments (Willkens et al., 1968), during the response of sensitized animals, synthesis of antigammaglobulin rheumatoid-like molecules can be detected.

Experimental arthritis induced by different techniques

In this chapter some techniques of experimentally induced arthritis will be briefly described; they are based on the use of lysosomal membrane and articular cartilage.

Arthritis can be induced by lysosomal enzymes in two different ways: (a) by using polymorphonuclear extracts, whose granules contain a large amount of lysosomal enzymes (Weissmann et al., 1967; Muirden and Phillips, 1973); and (b) by injecting intradermally or intra-articularly antibiotics, which, because of their high content of double links (filipin, etruscomycin etc.), cause the release of these enzymes. Interesting cases of experimental arthritis, in which alteration of the synovial membrane (synovial cell proliferation, infiltration of mononuclear and lymphoid cells) is associated with erosive action of a pannus on the articular cartilage, can be obtained.

The use of formalin, an arthritogenic substance, was suggested by Patrono in 1951; many authors (Scheiffarth et al., 1970) have used it since. The lesions obtainable are of short duration and therefore lack the feature of chronicity required for a reasonably good working model.

Among the arthritogenic substances carrageenan should be mentioned (Uruchurtu Marroquin and Ajmal, 1970); it is injected intra-articularly into swine.

A picture of synovitis (not arthritis) can be obtained with iron dextran injected parenterally in adult rabbits. When the experiment is carried out in young rabbits, in addition to the lesion already mentioned, a striking change in the chondrocytes of the articular cartilage, with fragmentation and 'slicing' of the cartilage surface, occurs.

Jasmin (1966) demonstrated that intravenous or intraperitoneal injection (in one single dose) of exudate from lymphosarcoma of Murphy resulted in a typical inflammatory polyarthritis in rats, with swelling of joints and histological signs of synovitis with lympho-mononuclear cells.

Recently Miller et al. (1970) presented a new model with which it is possible to obtain contemporaneously a picture of arthritis and inflammatory periarthritis using a subcutaneous injection of 6-sulfanilamidoindazole in adult rats. The articular and periarticular lesions are characterized by proliferative changes (not suppurative), with a large amount of lymphoid infiltrate. This type of arthritis is also of short duration.

The last model worth mentioning is the one suggested by Graham and Linpert Shannon (1972): with horse-radish peroxidase they observed a rheumatoid-like synovitis with plasma cells synthesizing antiperoxidase antibodies.

Conclusion

The attempt to correlate every type of experimental model of arthritis with a given human articular disease, which has been the basis of the continuous effort of many authors in recent years, cannot be considered unreasonable. The main difficulties can be summarized as follows:

1. The difficulty of correlating the lifespan of a given experimental animal with man;
2. The existence of a high degree of differences within species;
3. The difficulty of determining the self-perpetuating factors that could make the animal pathology easily resemble the human one;
4. The interference of genetic factors in the animals in comparison with man.

In our experience, in the field of immunological techniques, the most interesting models were the adjuvant and fibrin arthritis one in rabbits (according to the scheme of Dumonde and Glynn) and the model first carried out by Lucherini in the rhesus monkey. The latter has the advantage of acting as a long term process, with interesting evidence of delayed hypersensitivity which provide close parallels with human rheumatoid arthritis.

References

ANDREIS, M., STASTNY, P. and ZIFF, M. (1975): Experimental arthritis produced by injection of mediators of delayed hypersensitivity. *Rheumatology, 6*, 303.

BACON, F. A., BLUESTONE, R. and GOLDBERG, L. S. (1974): Experimental herpes virus arthritis factors in chronicity. *Ann. rheum. Dis., 33*, 413.

BARDEN, Y. A. and TULLY, Y. G. (1969): Experimental arthritis in mice with *Mycoplasma pulmonis. J. Bact., 100*, 5.

BAUMGARTNER, R., OBENAUS, H. and STOERK, H. C. (1974): Suppression of adjuvant arthritis by penicillamine in pyridoxine deficient rats. *Proc. Soc. exp. Biol., (N.Y.), 146*, 241.

BELOVIC, B. and KINSELLA, T. D. (1973): Immunofluorescent demonstration of an intra-articular antibody complex in experimental arthritis of the guinea pig. *Ann. rheum., Dis., 32,* 167.

BROUILHET, H., KAHAN, A., PIAITIER, D. and JOUANNEAU, M. (1975): Physiopathological aspect of Glynn's type of experimental arthritis. *Rheumatology, 6,* 308.

CARROZZO, M., POLLICE, L., SIMONE, C. and SIMPLICIO, F. (1972): Valutazione di alcuni parametri immunologici nell'artrite sperimentale del coniglio. *Folia allerg. (Roma), 19,* 21.

COLE, B. C., WARD, J. R., JONES, R. S. and CAHILL, J. F. (1971): Chronic proliferative arthritis of mice induced by *Mycoplasma arthitidis*. I. Induction of disease and histopathological characteristics. *Infect. Immun., 4,* 344.

CONSDEN, R., DOBLE, A., GLYNN, L. E. and NIND, A. (1971): The production of a chronic arthritis with ovalbumin and its retention in the rabbit knee joint. In: *Abstracts, VII European Rheumatology Congress,* 34/8.

COOK, Y., FINCHAN, W. Y. and LACK, C. H. (1969): Chronic arthritis produced by streptococcal L forms. *J. Path., 99,* 283.

DAVIS, B. (1971): Effects of prednisolone in an experimental model of arthritis in the rabbit. *Ann. rheum. Dis., 30,* 509.

DUMONDE, D. C. and GLYNN, L. E. (1962): The production of arthritis on rabbits by an immunological reaction to fibrin. *Brit. J. exp. Path., 43,* 373.

ENNIS, R. S., JOHNSON, J. S. and DECKER, J. L. (1972): Persistent *Mycoplasma hyorhinis* antigen in chronic mycoplasmal arthritis of swine. *Arthritis Rheum., 15,* 108.

GLYNN, L. E. (1975): The role of bacterial adjuvant in experimental arthritis. *Rheumatology, 6,* 283.

GRAHAM, R. C. and LINPERT SHANNON, S. (1972): Peroxidase arthritis. An immunologically mediated inflammatory response with ultrastructural cytochemical localization of antigen and specific antibody. *Amer. J. Path., 67,* 69.

HARWICK, H. J., KALMANSON, G. M., FOX, M. A. and GUZE, L. B. (1973a): Arthritis in mice due to infection with *Mycoplasma pulmonis*. I. Clinical and microbiological features. *J. infect. Dis., 128,* 533.

HARWICK, H. J., KALMANSON, G. N., FOX, M. A. and GUZE, L. B. (1973b): Mycoplasma arthritis of the mouse: development of cellular hypersensitivity to normal synovial tissue. *Proc. Soc. exp. Biol. (N.Y.), 144,* 561.

JASIN, H. E., COOKE, T. D. and HURD, E. R. (1973): Immunologic models used for the study of rheumatoid arthritis. *Fed. Proc., 32,* 147.

JASMIN, G. (1966): Experimental polyarthritis. *Laval Méd., 37,* 543.

KAPLAN, G. (1966): Problèmes posés par les polyarthrites expérimentales. *Sem. Hôp. Paris, 42,* 3183.

LAMAS DA SILVA, J. M. and ADLER, H. E. (1969): Pathogenesis of arthritis induced in chickens by *Mycoplasma gallisepticum*. *Pathol. Vet., 6,* 385.

LUCHERINI, T., CECCHI, E., PORZIO, F. and D'AMORE, A. (1965): Studi sulla provocazione di un'artrite sperimentale nel rhesus. *Minerva med., 56,* 323.

MALAGUZZI VALERI, C. and PIPITONE, V. (1972): Ricerche sull'attività immunodepressiva dell'indometacina. *Clin. ter., 61,* 293.

MALAGUZZI VALERI, C., PIPITONE, V., SCHIAVETTI, L. and PORZIO, F. (1971): Le artriti sperimentali. *Folia allerg. (Roma), 18,* 280.

MALAGUZZI VALERI, C., PIPITONE, V., SCHIAVETTI, L., PORZIO, F. and D'AMORE, A. (1972): Le artriti sperimentali. *Boll. Cent. Reum. Roma.*

MANSSON, I., NORBERG, R., OLHAGEN, B. and BJORKLUND, N. E. (1971): Arthritis in pigs induced by dietary factors. *Clin. exp. Immunol.*, 9, 677.

MARTIN, J. R., DE VRIES, J. and MOORE, S. (1968): Effect of papain on experimental E. coli infection. *Canad. med. Ass. J.*, 99, 68.

MILLER, M. L., WARD, Y. R., COLE, B. C. and SWINYARD, E. A. (1970): 6-Sulfanilamidoindazole induced arthritis and periarthritis in rats. A new model of experimental inflammation. *Arthritis Rheum.*, 13, 222.

MIZUSHIMA, Y., TSUKADA, W. and AKIMOTO, T. (1970): Prolongation of inflammation in rats inoculated with adjuvants. *Ann. rheum. Dis.*, 29, 178.

MOHN, S. F. and UTKLEV, H. E. (1970): Chronic polyarthritis in lambs caused by *Erysipelotrix insidiosa*. I. Clinical, pathologic and bacteriologic investigations. *Nord. Vet.-Med.*, 22, 236.

MOHR, W., WILD, A. and BENEKE, G. (1974): Chronische Osteomyelitis als Manifestation der Adjuvants-Krankheit der Ratte. *Beitr. Path.*, 153, 1.

MOWAT, A. G. and GARNER, R. W. (1972): Influence of iron dextran on adjuvant arthritis in the rat. *Ann. rheum. Dis.*, 31, 339.

MUIRDEN, R. D. and PHILLIPS, N. (1973): Evidence for a direct effect on articular cartilage and its lysosomal enzymes in filipin induced arthritis. *Ann. rheum. Dis.*, 32, 251.

NUMO, R., POLLICE, L., LAPADULA, G. and SCONOSCIUTO, C. (1975): Valutazione su parametri istologici ed immunitari di un modello di artrite nel coniglio con silicosi indotta. *Reumatismo*, in press.

NUMO, R., SALAMANNA, S., SIMONE, C. and SIMPLICIO, F. (1972): L'artrite sperimentale da fibrina nel coniglio: valutazione su parametri immunologici di una possibile azione immunodepressiva dell'indometacina. *Folia allerg. (Roma)*, 19, 195.

OCRA, P. L. and HERD, Y. K. (1971): Arthritis associated with induced rubella infection. *J. Immunol.*, 107, 810.

OLSON, N. O. and KERR, K. M. (1967): The duration and distribution of synovitis producing agents in chickens. *Avian Dis.*, 11, 578.

PEARSON, C. M. (1964): Experimental models in rheumatoid disease. *Arthritis Rheum.*, 7, 80.

PIERCY, D. W. (1970): Synovitis induced by intrarticular inoculation of inactivated *Mycoplasma mycoides* in calves. *J. comp. Path.*, 80, 549.

PIERSON, R. E. (1967): Polyarthritis in Colorado feedlot lambs. *J. Amer. vet. Med. Ass.*, 150, 1487.

RAWSON, A. Y., QUISMORIO, F. P. and ABELSON, N. N. (1969): The induction of synovitis in the normal rabbit with Fab. *Amer. J. Path.*, 54, 95.

ROBERT, J. E., RAMSEY, F. K. and SWITZER, W. P. (1968): Pathologic changes of porcine suppurative arthritis produced by *Streptococcus equisimilis*. *Amer. J. vet. Res.*, 29, 253.

SCHEIFFARTH, F., BAENKLER, H. W. and SCHOY, G. (1970): Wirkung und Speicherung von Gold bei der experimentallen Formalin-Arthritis der Ratte. *Z. Rheumaforsch.*, 23, 42.

SIKES, D. (1968): Experimental production of rheumatoid arthritis of swine; physiopathologic changes of tissues. *Amer. J. vet. Dis.*, 29, 1719.

SMITH, D. E., JAMES, P. G., SCHACHTER, J., ENGLEMAN, E. P. and MEYER, K. F. (1973): Experimental bedsonial arthritis. *Arthritis Rheum.*, 16, 21.

SOKOLOFF, L. (1973): Animal model. Arthritis due to Mycoplasma in rats and swine. *Amer. J. Path.*, 73, 261.

STEFFEN, C. and WICK, G. (1971): Delayed hypersensitivity reactions to collagen in rats with adjuvant induced arthritis. *Z. Immun. Forsch. Allerg. klin. Immun.*, 141, 169.

STEINBERG, M. E., McGRAW, C. R., COHEN, L. D. and SCHUMACHER, H. R. (1973): Pathogenesis of antigen induced arthritis. *Clin. Ortop.*, 97, 248.

TAYLOR, A. G., LACK, C. H. and FINCHAM, W. J. (1972): Synovitis produced by intra-articular injections of a non-haemolytic fraction of streptolysin-S preparations. *J. Path.*, *108*, 199.

TAYLOR, G., TAYLOR ROBINSON, D. and SLAVIN, G. (1974): Effect of immunosuppression on arthritis in mice induced by *Mycoplasma pulmonis*. *Ann. rheum. Dis.*, *33*, 376.

TIMONEY, J. F. and BERMAN, D. T. (1970): Erysipelothrix arthritis in swine: bacteriologic and immunopathologic aspects. *Amer. J. vet. Dis.*, *31*, 1411.

URUCHURTU MARROQUIN, A. and AJMAL, M. (1970): Carragenin induced arthritis in the specific pathogen free pig. *J. comp. Path.*, *80*, 607.

VOLKMAN, A. and COLLINS, F. M. (1973): Polyarthritis associated with Salmonella infection in rats. *Infect. Immun.*, *8*, 814.

WEBB, F. W., BLUESTONE, R. and GOLDBERG, L. S. (1973): Experimental viral arthritis induced with *Herpes simplex*. *Arthritis Rheum.*, *16*, 241.

WEISSMANN, G., BECHER, B., WIEDERMANN, G. and BERNHEIMER, A. W. (1965): Studies on lysosomes. VII. Acute and chronic arthritis produced by intra-articular injections of streptolysin S in rabbits. *Amer. J. Path.*, *46*, 129.

WEISSMANN, G., PRAS, N. and ROSENBERG, L. (1967): Arthritis induced by filipin in rabbits. *Arthritis Rheum.*, *10*, 325.

WHITEHOUSE, N. W., WHITEHOUSE, D. J., PETER, J. B. and PEARSON, C. M. (1971): Role of lymphocytes in rat adjuvant-induced arthritis and other autoallergic states: a clue to human therapeutics. In: *Abstracts, VII European Rheumatology Congress*, 34/4.

WILLKENS, R. F., ANDERSON, R. V. and GILLILAND, B. C. (1968): Response of sensitised rabbit to intra-articular gamma globulin. *Arthritis Rheum.*, *11*, 418.

ZIDEK, A. and PERLIK, F. (1971): Genetic control of adjuvant-induced arthritis in rats. *J. Pharm. Pharmacol.*, *23*, 389.

Chronopharmacology of anti-rheumatic drugs with special reference to indomethacin

E. C. Huskisson

Department of Rheumatology, St. Bartholomew's Hospital, London, United Kingdom

Chronopharmacology is concerned with the time course of the action of drugs. It is also concerned with the effect which the time of day at which a drug is given will have upon its actions. Indomethacin is an excellent example of a compound whose effects are greatly modified by the time of day at which it is given.

It is essential to know the time course of the action of a drug both for practical treatment of patients and for designing clinical trials. A drug which takes a few days to work, and which hasn't worked at the end of a week should be stopped before it has time to do some harm. Equally it is foolish to stop at the end of a week a drug which takes several months to produce an effect. In trials it is necessary to measure the effects of a drug at a time when those effects are maximal. This applies as much to unwanted effects of drugs as to the desired action. Side effects often occur at characteristic times during the course of a particular treatment and routine surveillance of patients should take this into consideration. In trials, the duration of treatment may enormously influence the incidence of side effects. A side effect which occurs after 6 months' treatment will not be detected in trials lasting 3 months.

The time course of the action of the different classes of anti-rheumatic drugs is illustrated in Figure 1. Simple analgesics such as paracetamol or aspirin in small doses act within about 30 minutes and their action lasts for about 6 hours. A second dose reproduces exactly the effects of the first. Measurement of this

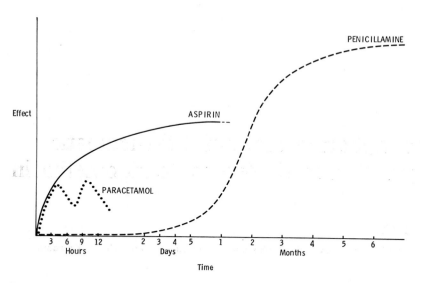

Fig. 1. The time course of the action of simple analgesics, anti-inflammatory drugs and drugs like penicillamine.

effect must therefore be made about 2 or 3 hours after administration if the effect is to be detected. Measurements made at other times, for example after a week of multiple doses may fail to detect any difference between an active drug and placebo. Anti-inflammatory drugs in general take a few days to reach their maximal effect. Measurements made at the end of a week are therefore satisfactory for most drugs and there is little point in waiting longer. Drugs with a specific action in rheumatoid arthritis, such as penicillamine, take 6 months to produce their maximal effect and again, measurement must be made at this time.

Penicillamine provides a most striking example of the relationship between the duration of treatment and the incidence of side effects (Balme and Huskisson, 1975). For example, proteinuria occurs only after 4 months' treatment and it is at this time that appropriate tests should be made. It is desirable to recognise the difference between two kinds of rashes, one occurring within a few weeks and easy to treat, another occurring after at least 6 months and usually requiring treatment to be stopped. The gastric side effects of aspirin are most likely to occur within the first month.

The beneficial effects of a large dose of indomethacin at night were first shown by Holt and Hawkins (1965) using the 100-mg suppository. Later Huskisson et al. (1970) compared administration by mouth and rectum. Huskisson and Hart (1972) compared indomethacin, aloxiprin and placebo, and Huskisson and Grayson (1974) compared indomethacin and sodium amylobarbitone. Though the rate of absorption is a little slower following oral administration, the effectiveness is a little greater. The effects of indomethacin at night are seen at a time when blood levels have fallen to a low level, peak levels occurring between 1 and 3 hours after administration depending on the route of administration. Indomethacin is superior to placebo, aloxiprin and sodium amylobarbitone. Three components of the response can be distinguished: there is relief of pain, reduction in the severity and duration of morning stiffness and improvement in the quality of sleep. Figure 2 (from Huskisson and Hart, 1972)

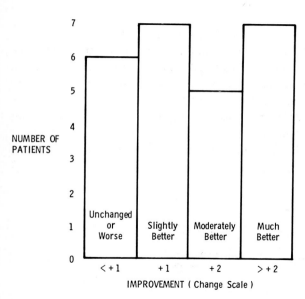

Fig. 2. Distribution of responses to indomethacin at night.

shows that about half of the patients treated were either moderately or much better. This was defined as a good response and it can be seen from Table 1 that this is most likely to occur in patients with morning stiffness lasting at least 30 minutes.

A further experiment was carried out to study the duration of the effect of indomethacin and to compare a large dose at night and a large dose in the morning. Ten patients with rheumatoid arthritis, all of whom were receiving regular night-time indomethacin, took part in the study. The duration of morning stiffness and 2-hourly pain scores (visual analogue scale) were measured

TABLE 1

*Influence of the duration of morning stiffness on the response to
indomethacin at night*

	Poor response	Good response
Morning stiffness		
> 30 minutes	5	10
< 30 minutes	8	2

$\chi^2 = 5.2$; $p < 0.05$

A good response was defined as moderately or much better on a pain relief scale, compared to placebo. (From Huskisson and Hart, 1972.)

for 4 consecutive days. Treatments were indomethacin at night as usual, no indomethacin, indomethacin at night as usual and indomethacin taken in the morning instead of at night. The results are shown in Figures 3, 4 and 5. The effect of indomethacin at night lasts until 4 p.m. the following day. Indomethacin at night is superior to indomethacin in the morning except in the late evening. Indomethacin taken in the morning does not reduce morning stiffness. Relief of pain is seen particularly in the second half of the day. Five patients experienced

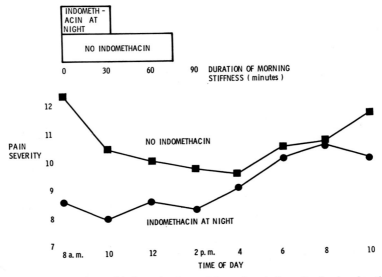

Fig. 3. Comparison of indomethacin at night and no indomethacin showing the duration of the effect.

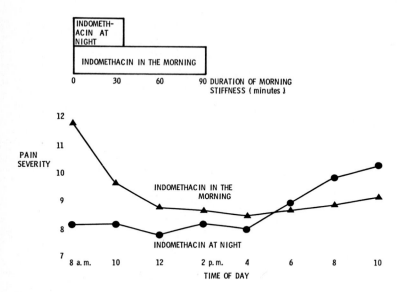

Fig. 4. Comparison of indomethacin at night with the same dose taken in the morning.

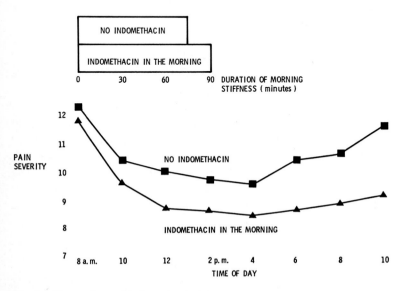

Fig. 5. Comparison of indomethacin in the morning and no indomethacin.

central nervous system side effects after taking indomethacin in the morning, sometimes severe; 1 patient had such side effects after taking indomethacin at night.

Data taken from Huskisson et al. (1970), an experiment in which 4 consecutive night-time doses of indomethacin were given, shows that the effect of this treatment is achieved on the first day and is not increased on the second and subsequent days (Figure 6).

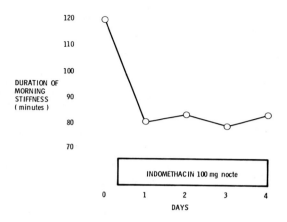

Fig. 6.   Response to indomethacin given for 4 consecutive nights showing that the full effect is achieved on the first night.

The following conclusions can be drawn and should be applied to the therapeutic use of indomethacin. If it doesn't work after the first administration of a large dose at night, it won't work and shouldn't be continued. It is most likely to work in patients with morning stiffness lasting at least 30 minutes. Administration at night is much more effective than administration in the morning and is less likely to cause side effects. The effects of a large dose of indomethacin in the morning are slight – it is probably better to reserve indomethacin for night-time use and use something else for the day. The time course of the effect of indomethacin suggests that it could be administered twice daily to produce pain relief throughout the day.

References

BALME, H. W. and HUSKISSON, E. C. (1975): Chronopharmacology of penicillamine and gold. *Scand. J. Rheumatol., Suppl. 8*, 21–07.

HOLT, P. J. L. and HAWKINS, C. F. (1965): Indomethacin: studies of absorption and of the use of suppositories. *Brit. med. J.*, *1*, 1354.

HUSKISSON, E. C. and GRAYSON, M. F. (1974): Indomethacin or amylobarbitone sodium for sleep in rheumatoid arthritis, with some observations on the use of sequential analysis. *Brit. J. clin. Pharmac.*, *13*, 176.

HUSKISSON, E. C. and HART, F. D. (1972): The use of indomethacin and aloxiprin at night. *Practitioner*, *208*, 248.

HUSKISSON, E. C., TAYLOR, R. T., BURSTON, D., CHUTER, P. J. and HART, F. D. (1970): Evening indomethacin in the treatment of rheumatoid arthritis. *Ann. rheum. Dis.*, *29*, 393.

Drug evaluation in rheumatoid arthritis

Norman O. Rothermich

Ohio State University, Columbus Medical Center Research Foundation, Columbus, Ohio, U.S.A.

No disease in the entire field of rheumatology provokes more controversy regarding drug effectiveness than rheumatoid arthritis. One can find strong support for the contention that rheumatoid arthritis is a very difficult disease to evaluate because of its marked day-to-day variations in intensity, because of its tendencies to spontaneous remissions and exacerbations and because of the commonly accepted belief that psychic or emotional factors exert strong influences on the evaluation of drug therapy. On the other hand, one could make just as good a case that rheumatoid arthritis is the easiest to evaluate because of the many parameters which allow more or less precise measurement of effect. For example, the disappearance of signs of active inflammation in a rheumatoid joint is much more readily discernible and measurable than the disappearance of pain in an osteoarthritic hip. Indeed, such things as the painful shoulder (whether it be bursitis, capsulitis, peri-arthritis or whatever name) are virtually impossible to subject to double-blind controlled studies.

In dealing with the problem of evaluation of drug efficacy in rheumatoid arthritis, certain principles must be established. The first basic is that rheumatoid arthritis does not lend itself to short-term studies. Pilot studies of 3, 6 or even 12 weeks may be of value in providing introductory, basic information about a drug, but no conclusions regarding therapeutic benefit should be drawn until a patient has been on a drug for a minimum of 6 months and preferably 12–24 months. As an example, my original studies on indomethacin were not reported until I had observed some patients on continuous treatment for 3 years or more. It was for that reason especially that I could feel confident of the validity of my conclusions.

The second principle, a belief of mine which may not be shared by others, is that every new drug study should involve crossover. Parallel studies alone can lead to fallacious conclusions. In our present state of knowledge we must assume that rheumatoid arthritis may not be a single disease entity. If there are indeed several different syndromes of rheumatoid arthritis, each may have different responsiveness to therapy. Since at present we have no way of distinguishing these different syndromes we may inadvertently load a parallel study in one direction or another by placing the majority of type A disease on the trial drug and most of the type B rheumatoid arthritis patients on the placebo.

As yet, no single agent (except cortisone) has been found to be effective in every case of rheumatoid arthritis; usually no more than 50 to 75% are benefitted, and remissions are far less frequent. Only by the use of placebo controls with crossover in all cases can we determine the true percentages and degrees of benefit in a new drug trial.

Furthermore, the problem of revealing side effects of any new drug is always present in any study. Almost every drug presently in use has some marker by which some patients can identify it. The percentage of such patient identification has to be determined and this can only be done by the use of placebo crossover. For example, we know that 20% or more of individuals experience revealing (though not necessarily serious) side effects from aspirin, such as gastric upset, heartburn, tinnitus, and even constipation. If we were to study aspirin as a new, wholly unknown drug in a parallel study, we might by chance have most of the side effects detectors in the placebo group. We would then be unaware of these various revealing side effects. On the other hand, if all of these individuals were in the active drug group, the incidence of such side effects might seem prohibitive. Parallel studies undoubtedly have some value, but cannot provide the wealth of information obtained from crossover studies.

Another principle is that double-blind controlled studies are not per se the total answer. In fact, I question whether any patient should be exposed for the first time to any new drug by entering immediately into a double-blind study. When patients are asked to participate in an experiment with a new and unknown drug they are naturally sensitized and over-alert to the possible hazards involved. It would be better to preface the double-blind study with a short period of open trial of the drug. In that way, patients will become more casual in the taking of the drug and the natural fears of catastrophic adverse effects or sudden death will be mitigated.

Although not customarily done, it may be advantageous to have patients on 'open trial' of an experimental drug for 4–8 weeks, before entering them into a double-blind controlled crossover trial. At the conclusion of the latter, the experiment should be continued on a single-blind basis with repeated inter-jection of placebo, especially in patients with uncertain degrees of benefit, or who have side effects questionably related to the experimental drug.

Another principle in new drug development is the need to establish with reasonable certainty that a given side effect is truly the result of the experimental drug, and not a coincidental happening. The literature on drugs (notably the package inserts and the 'PDR') has become cluttered with warnings, contra-indications, dangers and so forth, so voluminous that the practicing physician may overlook or not be aware of the few serious side effects which are really important and even a threat to the patient's life. Wherever it is possible and within the bounds of human ethics, every attempt should be made to reproduce an adverse effect in the same patient with the same drug. It is in this connection that single-blind placebo studies can yield their most important information. Few can deny that even the most astute investigator or clinician is susceptible to the specious reasoning of *post hoc ergo propter hoc*. Likewise the high inci-dence of adverse effects from placebo administration is well known. Therefore, the clear demonstration of causal relationship between the new drug and the adverse effect is imperative to both scientific and practical medicine. Too often, patients are denied potentially great benefits of a certain drug simply because of a reported side effect that was not sufficiently well documented.

In any new drug evaluation, there must be a balancing of and a weighing (as on the scales of justice) of the frequency and degree of benefit against the frequency and severity of side effects. Each scientist, each practicing physician and even each layman will view new drug data in a different light and from a different perspective. Those of us in the field of rheumatology, who deal with large numbers of cases of rheumatoid arthritis, have come to regard this disease as one of man's most vicious, painful and crippling, and are more willing to accept high rates of adverse side effects, if high rates and degrees of benefit can be obtained. I have often posed the hypothetical question: 'If a new drug were to be developed which could produce *cure*, in *every* case of rheumatoid arthritis, what would be an acceptable mortality for this drug?' This is not a simple rhetorical question but gets to the crux of the whole problem. For a layman who knows nothing whatsoever about the disease and has never had any con-tact with it, the answer might be 'zero'. However, to a deeply concerned rheuma-tologist, the answer might be as much as 4 or 5%, whereas to the individual afflicted with devastating progressive crippling disease, a mortality of 10 or 15% might be acceptable for a drug that would produce cure. These consider-ations are of paramount importance to developing the proper perspective on any new drug evaluation.

As indicated previously, new drug evaluation in rheumatoid arthritis may be at once very easy or very difficult and capricious, and therefore protocol studies are highly desirable. Criteria must be established at the outset and these must be followed as rigidly as possible. It has been well stated by Hart and his group from England as well as numbers of others that criteria that are most reliable are at the same time largely subjective. Under the pressure of statisticians we try to quantitate various criteria, but quite often we are simply quantitating patients' subjective responses, a classic example being duration of early morning stiffness. Rheumatologists know only too well how difficult it is to get a patient to give intelligent, consistent, knowledgeable answers with respect to early morning stiffness. Nevertheless, for want of something better we must continue this sort of thing, being always mindful of the subjective nature of the quantitation and not allowing statistical treatment to delude us.

I think we can all agree that there is no sacred formula, no sine qua non, no holier than thou message for evaluating drug efficacy in rheumatoid arthritis. Each investigator must establish his own criteria, conforming as much as possible to those criteria used by most other rheumatologists. It is important that he become thoroughly familiar with the criteria he proposes to use, and be consistent and objective in applying these criteria in the same way from patient to patient and from one new drug trial to another.

Our group at the Columbus Medical Center Research Foundation has developed a set of criteria which we believe fulfills our needs and gives us a reliable and dependable base for determining therapeutic efficacy. We have, for the sake of completeness and conformity, recorded other parameters in which we have less faith but we record them faithfully nevertheless. I will set forth here the 7 criteria which we have come to use and rely on heavily. We recognize that these 7 criteria in some respects can be quite harsh and often times we have found ourselves classifying a patient as unimproved on a certain drug because he failed to meet a sufficient number of these criteria, even though we may be convinced in our minds that the patient has had clinical benefit. These criteria are enumerated and explained as follows (Fig. 1):

1. Elimination of synovitis in all joints except one major *or* three minor joints. Active synovitis is revealed by joint swelling, pain on motion, but especially tenderness, and heat if present.

2. Elimination of nocturnal pain. We are of the opinion that nearly all patients with active rheumatoid arthritis are awakened during the night once, twice, and sometimes 5 or 6 times with pain of a rheumatic nature, usually associated directly with joints. We believe the elimination of all nocturnal rheumatic pain can be an important and reliable criterion.

3. Reduction of early morning stiffness to less than 30 minutes. If the initial

duration of early morning stiffness were only 30 minutes, then the reduction must be to 15 minutes or less.

4. Reduction of sedimentation rate by 50% of the original. We regard the sedimentation rate as the ultimate indicator of active rheumatoid inflammation. There are many other so-called 'acute phase reactants' which provide the same information but the sedimentation rate is so simple and so inexpensive that it is much preferred to any other. We are well aware that any tissue-destructive disease can influence the sedimentation rate, and this has to be taken into account in evaluating its variations.

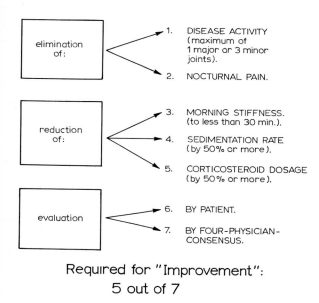

Required for "Improvement":
5 out of 7

Fig. 1. Therapeutic criteria.

5. The reduction by 50% of the required corticosteroid dosage. The dramatic effect of corticosteroid on the rheumatoid disease process is well known. Many of our more severe cases are on maintenance low-dosage corticosteroids usually prednisone, 5 mg or less, but never exceeding 10 mg as the total daily dose. The patient with rheumatoid arthritis becomes so dependent on the beneficial effects of even this small amount of corticosteroid that the ability to reduce the total daily dose by 50% becomes a valid and useful criterion.

6. The patient's evaluation of the benefit derived from an experimental drug is a criterion which can be of critical importance. In fact, the purists, the ultra-

scientific and the statisticians to the contrary notwithstanding, this may be the most important criterion of all.

7. The last of our criteria is the global evaluation by the physician. We try to make this a consensus evaluation of all 4 physicians in our group wherever this is possible and feasible, respecting, of course, the primacy of the attending physician's opinion. This global evaluation should not be just a summarization by the physician of the first 5 criteria but rather, he should exercise his clinical judgment regarding such things as the patient's sense of well-being, improvement of appetite, loss of toxic feelings, increase in activities of daily living, and increase in stamina throughout the day.

We have arbitrarily required that 5 of these criteria be fulfilled in order for a patient to be considered improved. All 7 must be affirmative if the patient is to be considered in remission (including absence of any synovitis).

It may be noted that I have not mentioned other commonly used criteria (Fig. 2). Most of these we carry out but feel that they are not as dependable

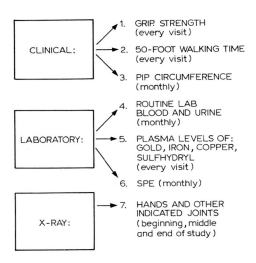

Fig. 2. Supplemental measures.

and consistent. For example, measurement of finger joint size can vary with time of day, the amount of usage of the hands and other factors. Walking time depends also on time of day, on motivation of the patient and other factors as well.

In summary, I have tried to point out certain general principles of new drug trials in the treatment of rheumatoid arthritis. Some of the aspects of these principles are philosophic but nevertheless are important to the clinical investigator. The actual manner in which we approach the problem of new drug evaluation has been described. I do not contend that ours is the sole (or the best) method, but in our hands we have found it practical and reliable.

Assessment of drug action in ankylosing spondylitis

F. Dudley Hart

24 Harmont House, 20 Harley Street, London, United Kingdom

Of all the patients who have cooperated with me in the assessments of drug action I place patients with ankylosing spondylitis very high. They have assisted in the assessment in the late 40's of deep X-ray therapy, in the early 50's of corticotrophins and different corticosteroids in the control of their disease, and also of phenylbutazone and oxyphenbutazone and in the 60's indomethacin and since then several other new compounds. These patients are usually good witnesses and not liable to placebo or nocebo reactions. They have high normal pain thresholds, are young and want to get on with life and the living of it. For out-patient trials they are usually excellent for their disease is much less prone to the swings of exacerbation and remission that are seen in rheumatoid arthritis. Also, over the last 30 years they have been excellent attenders in the clinic. Their only drawback in long-term studies is that, usually being young, they tend to move about the world more, emigrating to the U.S.A., Canada, Australia, New Zealand; annoyingly anywhere outside the London area and southern England. When the deep X-ray-leukaemia study was on, with the assistance of Sir Richard Doll and his department, we were nevertheless able to contact over 300 of 400 patients who had received this form of therapy. Incidently only one of those contacted had developed leukaemia.

Assessment methods

The patient is asked to record daily his pain and stiffness numerically and his morning stiffness in minutes (the limbering-up time). We have used the Dunham spondylometer (Dunham, 1949) in measuring spinal flexion and extension (Sturrock et al., 1973): it is a rapid and effective measure. Reynolds (1975) found it better than the commonly used Schober's skin distraction method (1937), though Loebl's inclinometer had certain advantages. Chest expansion at nipple level is measured in cm with hands on the head to avoid muscle contraction adding 2 cm or more to the figure (Moll and Wright, 1972). Assessments of sedimentation rate are useless as a measure of progress: seldom do they change significantly and then seldom in parallel with other measurements. Assessments of respiratory function may help, vital capacity in particular, care being taken to allow for apparent shortening in the patient's height from kyphosis due to the disease (Hart et al., 1963). Of all modes of assessment probably the best is the patient's own assessment of pain and stiffness and limbering-up times. Spinal range of movement, as assessed by photographic records, has not been particularly helpful, though spondylometry has helped in some trials (Sturrock and Hart, 1974). In the course of 30 years of assessment of these patients we have not found the steady progressive decline in spinal function or posture we were led to expect before the war. In a 20-year follow-up of 27 patients (Hart et al., 1974) where spinal range of movement was repeatedly measured, in only 8 was there progressive deterioration, 14 having measurements as good as, or better than, their assessment 10 to 26 years previously at their initial attendance.

Finally we have assessed function and position after surgical operations designed to improve posture or function. Lumbar spinal wedge osteotomy rarely needs to be done now, but it has improved both posture and function in the past. Mr. Charles Drew, F.R.C.S., cardio-thoracic surgeon to Westminster Hospital tried to improve intercostal movement by removing segments of the upper 5–7 ribs on each side. Improvement in respiratory function occurred for a time, then it returned to its previous state. Neck movements also improved at the time. He has now abandoned this operation.

The aim of all therapy in ankylosing spondylitis is to ease pain and improve function so that the patient can perform his daily exercises and do his daily duties at work and at home as fully and as freely as possible. This active kinetic approach under cover of effective anti-inflammatory agents by day and by night has been a huge improvement on the bad old pre-war days of static immobility in plaster and other restrictive jackets and supports.

References

DUNHAM, W. F. (1949): *Brit. J. phys. Med.*, *12*, 126.
HART, F. D., EMERSON, P. A. and GREGG, I. (1963): *Ann. rheum. Dis.*, *22*, 11.
HART, F. D., STRICKLAND, D. and CLIFFE, P. (1974): *Ann. rheum. Dis.*, *33*, 136.
MOLL, J. M. H. and WRIGHT, V. (1972): *Ann. rheum. Dis.*, *31*, 1.
REYNOLDS, P. M. G. (1975): *Rheumat. Rehab.*, *14*, 180.
SCHOBER, P. (1937): *Münch. med. Wschr.*, *84*, 336.
STURROCK, R. D. and HART, F. D. (1974): *Ann. rheum. Dis.*, *33*, 129.
STURROCK, R. D., WOJTULEWSKI, J. A. and HART, F. D. (1973): *Rheumatol. and Rehabil.*, *12*, 135.

Non-steroidal anti-inflammatory agents in gout

Giampiero Pasero

Servizio di Reumatologia, University of Pisa and S. Chiara Hospital, Pisa, Italy

An evaluation of non-steroidal anti-inflammatory (NSAI) agents in the treatment of gout seems to be quite easy: their use in fact is rather limited. However, it may be desirable to clarify the limits of their utilization and what can be expected from these drugs in medical practice.

Semantically the term 'gout' has two separate meanings. Gout is a metabolic disorder, characterized by a probably non-univocal error of purine metabolism, resulting in an increase of urate miscible pool. Gout is also a clinical syndrome with well defined and typical acute distress, which may develop into a chronic, sometimes rheumatoid-like, arthritis. The gouty metabolic disorder usually induces the gouty clinical syndrome, but it may also remain asymptomatic for a long time or always. The gouty clinical syndrome is usually associated with the metabolic disorder, but any hyperuricemia can induce a 'secondary' gout.

The aim of the treatment of gout is therefore on the one hand to correct the metabolic defect, or at least to deplete the urate pool, and on the other to control the inflammatory response subsequent to the intra-articular deposition of urate crystals. The main indication for NSAI agents is obviously acute attack, but in particular cases they could also be used in the basic treatment of the disease.

NSAI agents in the treatment of acute gouty arthritis

In acute attack NSAI drugs represent the only true alternative to colchicine, since the usefulness of corticosteroids is of restricted value. Their fitness may be compared to that of colchicine (Kuzell et al., 1954; Ballabio et al., 1963): the effect is perhaps slightly delayed, but they are on the whole better tolerated. A proper comparative trial is however not easy to perform because the acute attack is naturally self-limited. The time-honoured preferences of many rheumatologists for colchicine is strengthened by the diagnostic value of its administration. Most cases of acute arthritis improve with indometacin or phenylbutazone, but, with the sole exception of sarcoid arthritis (Kaplan, 1963), only acute gouty arthritis is responsive to colchicine.

In order to better understand the mode of action of colchicine and NSAI agents, it is useful to summarize the pathogenesis of acute attack (Marmont et al., 1969). Precipitation of urate crystals in synovial fluid seems to be the starting event (McCarthy and Hollander, 1961), and intra-articular injection of a suspension of urate crystals, but not of amorphous urate or solution of urate, is capable of producing an inflammatory reaction even in non-gouty subjects. (Seegmiller et al., 1962). Urate crystals are liable to phagocytosis by synovial leukocytes and included in lysosomes, of which they labilize the membrane, with subsequent release of lysosomal hydrolases through cytoplasmic microtubules (McCarthy, 1963). On the other hand, the urate crystals free in synovial fluid activate Hageman factor with a subsequent 'cascade' activation of kallikrein and kinin systems (Marmont et al., 1969). Lysosomal enzymes and bradykinin are the most likely mediators of the inflammatory process induced by urate crystals. The role of prostaglandins has not yet been clarified, but seems of lesser importance than in other types of synovitis (Patrono and Bombardieri; unpublished data). It should however be recalled that prostaglandins sensitize the receptors to the action of bradykinin (Moncada et al., 1973) and that prostaglandin synthetase originates from lysosomes (Hamberg et al., 1974).

A series of vicious circles maintains this process: the cell death that follows the rupture of lysosomes releases urate crystals, which can be phagocytosed by other leukocytes; increased lactic acid production due to phagocytosis reduces synovial pH and urate solubility; new cells are attracted in the inflamed joint by chemotactic factors released by polymorphonuclear leukocytes after phagocytosis or through the activation of the complement pathway (Marmont et al., 1969). The autocatalytic nature of the inflammatory response to urate precipitation in synovial fluid fits with the clinical picture of acute gouty arthritis, i.e. the sudden onset and the unusually quick progression of inflammation and pain.

Colchicine interacts with tubulin, and becomes able to disrupt the assembly and function of cytoplasmic microtubules through which lysosomal enzymes disperse (Wilson et al., 1974); in a similar way the drug behaves as a poison of mitotic spindle (Borisy and Taylor, 1967). The mode of action of NSAI agents is still doubtful, although there is evidence that they inhibit some mediators of the inflammatory response, i.e. bradykinin (Collier and Shorley, 1960), or, according to recent opinion, prostaglandins (Vane, 1971).

NSAI agents in the basic treatment of gout

There is no doubt that basic treatment of gout should aim to deplete the urate miscible pool. The utilization of NSAI agents can be examined from several points of view.

First of all, it should be emphasized that urate pool depletion induces an indirect influence on the clinical picture. Only after a consistent depletion of the urate pool does the frequency of acute attacks decline and then subside. In contrast, the beginning of effectual urate-depleting therapy with uricosuric agents or allopurinol is often marked by an increased susceptibility to acute attacks (De Seze and Rychewaert, 1960), probably owing to urate mobilization from tissue deposits. Consequently, in the first few weeks or months of such treatment anti-inflammatory drugs are usually administered in order to prevent the possible worsening of the disease. In this respect NSAI drugs are preferred to colchicine, which is frequently associated with undesirable side effects.

Moreover, it has still to be established if urate-depleting therapy is sufficient to achieve long-term, complete remission of the clinical symptoms or if anti-inflammatory drugs can objectively contribute to a more complete recovery. In some cases chronic gouty arthritis closely resembles rheumatoid arthritis, so that the term 'gouty rheumatism' has been suggested (Coste and Delbarre, 1956). I do not think that this term helps to clarify the matter: a gouty polyarthritis can mimic a rheumatoid arthritis from which, however, it can easily be distinguished (Pasero and Riccioni, 1962), at least owing to its sensitivity to urate-depleting therapy. Undoubtedly it is not easy to obtain long-term, practically unlimited, urate-depleting treatment in all patients, so that periodically it may be necessary to use NSAI agents; however, I do not feel that the omission of a more efficacious therapy may strictly represent an indication for a drug. On the other hand it is very doubtful whether there exists a variety of chronic gouty arthritis in which the inflammation is so independent from urate deposition as to persist after urate pool depletion.

NSAI agents and uric acid metabolism

NSAI drugs have different effects on serum uric acid levels, that are reduced by phenylbutazone (Kuzell et al., 1954), pyrasanone (Pasero and Ciompi, 1973) and high dosages of aspirin (Yu and Gutman, 1953), increased by aspirin below 2 g/day (Yu and Gutman, 1953), and unaffected by indometacin (Ballabio et al., 1963), phenamates (Latham et al., 1966) and ibuprofen (Loizzi et al., 1973).

Theoretically it would be possible to use some NSAI drugs in the basic treatment of gout with the dual aim of both controlling the urate pool and the inflammatory response. It is however not advisable to administer an unlimited amount of these drugs such as would be needed to mantain an effective depletion of the urate pool. It should be noted, nevertheless, that sulphinpyrazone, a phenylbutazone derivative devoid of significant anti-inflammatory properties is actually utilized in gout as a uricosuric agent (Persellin and Schmid, 1961).

The mechanism of the urate-depleting properties of some NSAI agents is not yet completely clarified. Since reduction of serum uric acid is associated with increased urate renal excretion, it is generally believed that these drugs act through inhibition of tubular reabsorption of urate. The non-univocal effect of aspirin has been cited to suggest a double mechanism of urate tubular handling: a secretory one, more sensitive to aspirin, and a reabsorptive one, only sensitive to higher doses of the drug (Yu and Gutman, 1953). The binding of phenylbutazone to plasma proteins, which could compete with that of urate may account for increased urate filtration (Bluestone et al., 1970). Indometacin also binds strongly with plasma proteins (Kucera and Bullock, personal communication), but lacks any effect on serum uric acid; most likely the displacing effect of different drugs on protein-bound urate depends on the binding site and avidity of ligands. Binding of indometacin to serum albumin, for instance, can be displaced by salicylic acid, but not by phenylbutazone or probenecid (Yesair et al., 1970). Furthermore, phenylbutazone reduces serum uric acid more than it increases urate renal excretion; this can be accounted for by the haemodilution due to the salt-retaining activity of the drug or, alternatively, by redistribution of uric acid between the intra- and extravascular pools, due to the displacing effect of the drug urate-protein binding (Pasero and Ciompi, 1973). The latter hypothesis may explain the induction of gouty attacks in patients started on phenylbutazone (Pasero and Ciompi, 1973).

The urate-depleting effect of some NSAI drugs may parallel the anti-inflammatory activity of some uricosuric agents. Phenylquinoline-carbonic acid, a drug no longer used because of its hepatotoxicity, shared both urate-depleting and anti-inflammatory activity. Some years ago, while studying the uricosuric activity of 5-bromophenyl-indanedione, we noticed that none of the gouty patients started on this drug complained of acute attacks at the beginning of the treatment (Pasero and Riccioni, 1963). Later 5-bromophenyl-indanedione was found to display anti-inflammatory properties similar to those of aspirin (Lombardino and Wiseman, 1968).

In view of the effect of some NSAI drugs on the serum uric acid level, in order to correctly evaluate the significance of this level, it is useful to ascertain if the patient is on treatment with these drugs, since uric acid level is usually requested in patients with joint complaints. Conversely, if a NSAI agent has to be given to a patient with a possible gouty arthritis, it is advisable to apply a drug, such as indometacin, devoid of any effect on the serum uric acid level.

References

BALLABIO, C. B., CIRLA, E., GIRARDI, G., CARUSO, I. and COLOMBO, B. (1963): Effetti clinici e metabolici dell'indomethacin nelle malattie reumatiche. *Reumatismo, 14*, 487.

BORISY, G. G. and TAYLOR, E. W. (1967): The mechanism of action of colchicine. Colchicine binding to sea urchin eggs and the mitotic apparatus. *J. Cell Biol., 34*, 535.

BLUESTONE, R., KIPPEN, I., KLINENBERG, J. R. and WHITEHOUSE, W. M. (1970): Factors affecting the binding of urate to plasma proteins. *Ann. rheum. Dis., 29*, 330.

COLLIER, H. O. J. and SHORLEY, P. G. (1960): Analgesic antipyretic drugs as antagonists of bradykinin. *Brit. J. Pharmacol., 15*, 601.

COSTE, F. and DELBARRE, F. (1956): Existe-t-il un rhumatisme gouttoux? *Méd. Hyg., 14*, 285.

DE SEZE, S. and RYCHEWAERT, A. (1960): *La Goutte.* Paris, Expansion Scientifique, Paris.

HAMBERG, M., SVENSSON, J. and SAMUELSSON, B. (1974): Prostaglandin endoperoxides. A new concept concerning the mode of action and release of prostaglandins. *Proc. nat. Acad. Sci. (Wash.), 71*, 3824.

KAPLAN, H. (1963): Further experience with colchicine in the treatment of sarcoid arthritis. *New Engl. J. Med., 268*, 761.

KUZELL, W. C., SCHAFFARZICK, R. W., NAUGLER, W. E., GAUDIN, G., MANKLE, E. A. and BROWN, B. (1954): Phenylbutazone (Butazolidin) in gout. *Amer. J. Med., 16*, 212.

LATHAM, B. A., RADCLIFF, F. and ROBINSON, R. G. (1966): The effect of mefenamic acid and flufenamic acid on plasma uric acid levels. *Ann. Phys. Med., 8*, 242.

LOIZZI, P., CARROZZO, M. and PIPITONE, V. (1973): Studio della clearance dell'acido urico correlata all'impiego di un farmaco antireumatico non steroideo. *Minerva Med., 64*, 2568.

LOMBARDINO, J. G. and WISEMAN, E. H. (1968): Anti-inflammatory 2-aryl-1,3-indanediones. *J. med. Chem., 11*, 342.

MARMONT, A., DAMASIO, E., ROSSI, F. et al. (1969): Alcuni aspetti patogenetici dell'attacco acuto di gotta. *Reumatismo, 21*, 152.

MCCARTHY JR, D., (1963): Crystal induced inflammation: syndromes of gout and pseudo-gout. *Geriatrics, 18*, 467.

MCCARTHY JR, D. and HOLLANDER, J. L. (1961): Identification of urate crystals in gouty synovial fluid. *Ann. Intern. Med., 54*, 452.

MONCADA, S., FERREIRA, S. H. and VANE, J. R. (1973): Prostaglandins, aspirin-like drugs and the oedema of inflammation. *Nature (Lond.), 246*, 217.

PASERO, G. and CIOMPI, M. L. (1973): Recherches sur l'action hypouricémiante de la pyrazino-butazone. In: *Symposium International sur L'inflammation Rheumatismale, p. 111.*

PASERO, G. and RICCIONI, N. (1962): Le artropatie uratiche atipoche nel quadro delle manifestazioni della gotta cronica. *Giorn. clin. Med. (Bologna)*, *43*, 283.

PASERO, G. and RICCIONI, N. (1963): Il 2-fenil-5-bromo-1,3-indandione nel trattamento uricurico della diatesi urica. *Clin. Ter.*, *26*, 32.

PERSELLIN, R. H. and SCHMID, F. R. (1961): The use of sulphinpyrazone in the treatment of gout. *J. Amer. med. Assoc.*, *175*, 971.

SEEGMILLER, J. E., HOWELL, R. R. and MALAWISTA, S. E. (1962): The inflammatory reaction to sodium urate. *J. Amer. med. Ass.*, *180*, 469.

VANE, J. R. (1971): Inhibition of prostaglandin synthesis as a mechanism of action for aspirin-like drugs. *Nature (Lond.)*, *231*, 232.

WILSON, L., BAMBURG, J. R., MIZEL, S. B., GRISHAM, L. M. and CRESWELL, K. M. (1974): Interaction of drugs with microtubule proteins. *Fed. Proc.*, *33*, 158.

YESAIR, D. W., REMINGTON, L., CALLAHAN, M. and KENSLER, C. J. (1970): Comparative effects of salicylic acid, phenylbutazone, probenecid and other anions on the metabolism, distribution and excretion of indomethacin by rats. *Biochem. Pharmacol.*, *19*, 1591.

YU, T. F. and GUTMAN, A. B. (1953): Paradoxical retention of uric acid by uricosuric drugs in low dosage. *Proc. Soc. exp. Biol. (N.Y.)*, *84*, 20.

Treatment of the acute painful shoulder by non-steroidal anti-inflammatory drugs

A. P. Peltier

Hôpital Lariboisière, Paris, France

Inflammation is one of the essential mechanisms of pain in the acute painful shoulder, whatever the anatomical structure affected and whatever the exact pathogenic mechanisms of these attacks may be. This accounts for the place of choice which anti-inflammatory drugs occupy amongst non-specific therapeutic measures that can be used in the majority of cases.

Evaluation of the efficacy of treatment

The general rules for estimating the efficacy of all treatments naturally apply here in the case of anti-inflammatory treatment. Among the factors that must be judged (Table 1), spontaneous pain, as well as the subjective element, remains one of the most important. The presence or absence of night pain is in this respect a major part of the evaluation. It should be defined if this pain is more or less permanent, connected with the position in bed, temporarily connected with leaning on the painful shoulder or with a certain position of the arm, disappearing when the position is changed. Only the first type of pain should be considered when judging the results of anti-inflammatory treatment.

When judging active and passive mobility, besides the classic movements of abduction and external rotation, the movement of internal rotation and retropulsion (the extent of which is measured by placing the hand as high as possible

TABLE 1

Evaluation of the efficacy of anti-inflammatory treatment in acute painful shoulder

---

Factors to be considered:

  I. Spontaneous pain (scaled from 0 to 4)

    0 = no pain,
    1 = slight pain,
    2 = moderate pain,
    3 = marked pain,
    4 = intense pain (very acute).

    To note at each examination:
    a. spontaneous pain during the day (average intensity);
    b. night pain (night before examination);
    c. pain on active movement.

  II. Local sensitivity: pain on palpation

    See spontaneous pain, scaled from 0 to 4.

 III. Extent of movements

    a. entire abduction (free shoulder blade);
    b. abduction of only the gleno-humerus (frozen shoulder blade);
    c. internal rotation and combined retropulsion (in cm);
    d. external rotation.

 IV. Overall judgment

    a. Subjective impression of patient: effect of medication: very good, good, average, debatable, nil.
    b. Opinion of clinician: same scale as above.

---

on the back to within a thumb's distance from C7 and compared with the good side) is of particular interest.

Results

Nearly 80% of acute painful shoulders are due to periarticular attacks which are included under the general term of scapulo-humeral periarthritis (SHP).

Painful shoulder (simple)

Painful shoulder (simple) is generally caused by tendinitis of the supraspinatous tendon, more rarely a tendinitis of the long biceps or of the infraspinatous. This tendinitis, simple degenerative or calcified, can become acutely painful due to mechanical (traumatic, overstress etc.) or climatic causes, or even without apparent reason. Besides the local infiltration of corticosteroids, analgesics and resting the shoulder, these conditions benefit greatly from anti-inflammatory drugs administered either in a relatively prolonged manner and in weak or average doses in simple form, or as brief treatment with large doses (injected) into the acute area. In certain cases, the pain and the functional problems persist for an abnormally long time and are resistant to anti-inflammatory agents and it is necessary to consider a rupture of the rotator cuff. In this instance, when suturing the ruptured cuff, it may be considered necessary to transpose externally the supraspinatous (or infraspinatous) tendon in order to stitch these tendons to the trochanter; otherwise it may only be a case of tendon calcification in which the incision itself may lead to a cure.

Pseudoparalytic shoulder

The pseudoparalytic shoulder caused by rupture of the rotator cuff can, at the moment it occurs, be accompanied by acute pain especially in severe traumatic forms. The anti-inflammatory and analgesic treatment will only have an effect on the initial pain: by contrast, it is of course without effect on the paralysis, which is pathognomonic of the rupture. If this paralytic weakness does not decline spontaneously after two or three months, it is necessary to consider a surgical repair of the affected tendons.

Acute hyperalgesic shoulder

The acute hyperalgesic shoulder is a genuine rheumatological emergency characterised by intense pain, making all movement of the shoulder impossible and entailing insomnia. Anatomically, it is caused by either an intense and very severe inflammation at the site of calcification of a tendon of the rotator cuff (a real tendinous 'boil'), or a migration of tendinous calcification in the serous sub-acromion-deltoid bursa, or, possibly, an acute exudative sub-acromion-deltoid bursitis. Here any local infiltration treatment can be very painful and the best treatment is that administered systematically, bringing the most rapid recession of the inflammatory process. Powerful anti-inflammatory agents such as phenylbutazone intramuscularly in a dosage of 600 mg/24 hours, or indometacin by mouth or by suppositories, at maximal dosage, offer a choice of treatments.

Retractable capsulitis

Retractable capsulitis, when first appearing, includes an inflammatory element which shows itself histologically as a discrete perivascular infiltration consisting of mononuclear cells embedded in a considerable fibrous thickening of the capsule. Anti-inflammatory drugs given by the usual method and in decreasing doses for six to eight weeks can control the pain at this stage of onset, but they are without effect at the stage of 'frozen shoulder', when only re-education over several weeks or months permits the restoration of normal mobility.

Attacks of true scapulo-humeral arthritis

Five to 15% of painful shoulders are caused by an attack of scapulo-humeral arthritis but by very varied processes: infectious, rheumatic, metabolic (chondrocalcinosis), degeneration (arthrosis), vascular (necrosis), nervous (arthropathy of the spinal cord), tumorous, etc. The exact therapeutic indications here depend essentially on the aetiology. Attacks caused by rheumatic pelvispondylitis or chondrocalcinosis are, for instance, excellent indications for non-steroidal anti-inflammatory agents.

Assessment of anti-inflammatory drugs in osteoarthritis of the hip and the knee

I. Caruso, F. Montrone and L. Carratelli

Ospedale L. Sacco and Servizio di Reumatologia, Milan, Italy

As yet no sure and reproducible method of assessment of osteoarthritis is available. No clinical or biological element has proved to be closely related to the course of the disease. Even the study of synovial fluid with the facilities now available to us failed to produce any 'marker' sufficiently sensitive to the clinical variations of the disease.

Nonetheless, a series of articular parameters mainly based on pain and function may provide adequate evaluation of the clinical stage of the disease and of the patient's degree of functional impairment. Radiology then enables us to discriminate the form and the stage of the degenerative joint process.

This paper will provide an example of a protocol for the clinical evaluation of osteoarthritis of the hip and the knee, two joints that are most suited for the use of the above-mentioned parameters. The main purpose of the protocol is to identify and to quantitate as far as possible the oscillations of activity of osteoarthritis and the effects of possible therapies. The protocol is made up of three parts. The first includes the questions aimed at identifying and classifying the form of disease from a pathogenetic, functional and radiological point of view. The second consists of the patient's assessment of his or her own osteoarthritic condition. The third is devoted to the investigator's assessment, based on the study of the function of the joint.

The form of disease

General data (weight, height, age, occupation) and all elements concerning the patient's history which may prove useful in identifying any general or local factors which predisposed, conditioned or determined the onset of osteoarthritis (such as dysplasias, traumas, metabolic disorders, etc.), are noted.

Particular emphasis is laid on the distinction between the primary and secondary forms of the disease, since they differ in terms of prognosis, evolution and therapeutic response. This distinction is not always easy to make. In principle, there are some elements which help to distinguish primary from secondary forms, i.e. early onset, symmetry of localization, symptoms of hyperalgesia.

In the hip-femur joint, the primary form is evidenced by the axial or lower polar pinching of the rima articularis; in the knee it is evidenced by the involvement of the femoro-patellar joint. Femoro-patellar osteoarthritis very often precedes femoro-tibial osteoarthritis. These forms indicate that the cartilage degeneration is unconnected with and independent of mechanical load factors, which, however, can affect the development and severity of the disease.

The first part of the protocol also includes the functional classification of osteoarthritis according to the A.R.A. criteria (Table 1) and the radiological evaluation according to an arbitrary scale ranging from 0 to 4, depending on the severity of radiological alterations (Table 2).

TABLE 1

Functional classification of osteoarthritis

Class I:	Possibility of accomplishing all normal activities without handicap.
Class II:	Possibility of accomplishing normal activities, despite the occurrence of pain or the articular impairment of one or more joints.
Class III:	Reduced occupational activity; reduced ability to care for oneself.
Class IV:	Strongly reduced occupational activity; patient keeping to bed or to a chair; reduced or nil ability to care for oneself.

TABLE 2

Radiological evaluation of osteoarthritis

0:	Normal.
1:	Slight reduction in the joint space.
2:	Reduction in the joint space, osteophytes, slight bone sclerosis.
3:	Marked reduction in the joint space, osteophytes, change in the bone structure.
4:	Disappearance of the joint space, sclerosis and cysts, large osteophytes and marked change in the bone structure.

Patient's evaluation

The second part of the protocol includes a series of questions for the patient, concerning his or her osteoarthritic condition. The answers may provide the investigator with a basis for judging the degree of impairment and pain. These questions are related to pain under load and on walking, night pain, and pain in the performance of specific activities, such as climbing up the stairs, getting out of bed or the bathtub, etc. (Table 3).

TABLE 3

Evaluation of the osteoarthritic condition by the patient

	Pain under load and/or in walking	Pain in the performance of specific activities	Night pain
Degree 0 Absence of pain	No interference with walking or with the upright position.	No interference in routine activities, such as climbing up the stairs, getting out of bed, etc.	No interference with sleep
Degree 1 Mild pain	Pain under load which disappears completely with rest.	No interference with the performance of routine activities.	Pain is only felt after waking up.
Degree 2 Moderate pain	Continuous pain, attenuated but not completely abolished with rest.	The patient has to make repeated attempts to accomplish activity.	The patient often wakes up because of pain.
Degree 3 Strong pain	Continuous pain, compelling the patient to stop action soon after starting.	The patient needs support in order to accomplish activity.	At times pain completely prevents sleep.
Degree 4 Severe pain	Impossible to stand up and walk without support.	Incapacity to accomplish activity, even with support.	Sleep is completely prevented by pain.

Investigator's assessment

This part of the protocol includes the investigator's assessment of the patient's osteoarthritic condition. It is based on the study of the excursions of joints in passive movements. The parameters to be taken into consideration are in our opinion the following: flexion, extra-intra-rotation, and abduction for the hip-femur joint; extension and flexion for the knee. All such measurements are expressed in degrees, apart from the abduction of the thigh bone, which is usually indicated in cm as intermalleolar distance.

The variations in these parameters as a result of therapy do not run parallel. In osteoarthritis of the hip with lower pinching of the rima articularis the flexion of the thigh may score a significant increase as a result of steroid infiltration, whereas abduction is barely modified or completely unchanged (Caruso, unpublished data). Hence the imperative need for all the above-mentioned parameters to be carefully evaluated. Abduction however is the easiest parameter to record and the least susceptible to errors of evaluation.

The assessment of osteoarthritis of the hip and of the knee based on all the data illustrated in the protocol may be considered as sufficiently objective and makes it possible for the various stages of the clinical course to be identified. The problems arise when these evaluations are used for clinical trials and therefore have to provide indications as to the changes in the disease's activity as induced by an analgesic-anti-inflammatory drug. The situation is further complicated when this judgement concerns the change induced by two drugs under comparison.

It is well known that pain is by far the most important parameter in suggesting and determining the global judgement of the investigator and the patient. Pain is the main cause of functional impairment for most of these patients and it is highly unlikely that, in the course of analgesic-anti-inflammatory therapy, a functional improvement would be observed without concurrent relief of pain. But pain is a purely subjective phenomenon resulting from a number of elements which elude any objective evaluation, so much so that the emotional component quite often turns out to predominate.

An example of the difficulties encountered in the evaluation of osteoarthritis of the hip and of the knee is provided by the results, still incomplete, of one of the most extensive multi-center research studies comparing two drugs, Sulindac and acetylsalicylic acid, under double-blind conditions. With the permission of Merck, Sharp and Dohme, we here report some of these data concerning the treatment of osteoarthritis of the hip and of the knee over a period of 24 weeks.

Table 4 shows that in the investigator's opinion there was a significant difference between the two drugs: the number of patients scoring an 'excellent + good' result was significantly higher among those treated with Sulindac. Sulindac also provided better results in the patient's opinion, but the difference in terms of results obtained with the two drugs was statistically significant only in the 4–8-week period. There was accordingly a discrepancy in the global evaluation of the osteoarthritic condition as made by a team of investigators and by a group of patients.

TABLE 4

Comparative trial with Sulindac (A) and acetylsalicylic acid (B) in osteoarthritis of hip and/or knee

Period	Treatment		Investigator's assessment	Patient's opinion
Week 4	A	215		
	B	193	+ +	N S
	Total	408		
Week 8	A	199		
	B	165	+ +	+
	Total	364		
Week 16	A	67		
	B	60	+	N S
	Total	127		
Week 24	A	31		
	B	25	+ +	N S
	Total	56		

+Statistically significant difference, $P < 0.05$.
++Statistically significant difference, $P < 0.01$.

The analysis of the individual parameters showed that both drugs modified the objective parameters concerning the joints in a superposable way, with statistically significant differences with respect to the original conditions. For the patient therefore, the variation in the subjective sensation of pain had more influence than any other parameter on his/her evaluation of his/her osteo-arthritic condition, and consequently of the activity of the drug. As for the investigator, on many occasions his less favourable judgement, apparently at odds with the objective data, was due to side effects, which proved to be statistically more frequent and serious with acetylsalicylic acid than with Sulindac.

Instrumental measurement of drug effects

U. Ambanelli

Servizio di Reumatologia, Istituto di Clinica Medica, University of Parma, Italy

The evaluation of the pharmacological properties of an anti-inflammatory agent is strictly dependent on a quantitative evaluation of the inflammation. For this reason, many rheumatologists have been engaged in studying experimental and clinical methods which could guarantee an objective evaluation of inflammation through a series of quantitative parameters. This was not possible with the traditional methods. However, the results achieved in this way are very far from representing an ideal solution of the problem. The ideal method should note one of the cardinal signs of inflammation (calor, tumor, rubor, dolor and functio laesa) (Pasero, 1975; Huskisson, 1974) (Table 1).

It is well known that inflamed joints are warmer than the surrounding tissue and that a thermographic study can evaluate the grade of inflammation of the joint. However, it is only recently that thermographic studies using telethermographs have been reported (Cosh and Ring, 1970; Collins et al., 1974; Ring and Collins, 1970; Ring et al., 1974; Haberman et al., 1971). The black and white thermographic technique shows the warmest areas as those with the greater intensity of gray, but it is extremely important to pay attention to some technical details; e.g. the room must be at a homogeneous and constant temperature, and the patient well adapted to this temperature. The same technique may be applied in colors. In this case the isometric areas are derived from the standards of the machine and from the chromatic scales usually reported in the same photograph reporting the result.

With these machines it is possible to demonstrate warm areas impeding on the joints clinically affected by inflammatory arthropathies. A good correlation

TABLE 1

Characteristics of the ideal method for evaluation of the anti-inflammatory properties of a therapeutic agent

---

Evaluation of a fundamental symptom:
  Objective
  Quick
  Standard:
    low variability of results for the same investigator
    low variability of results between different investigators

  Independent of external causes
  May be repeated shortly
  Not harmful
  In all the joints

Technique
  Sensitive
  Quantitative
  Not harmful for patient or investigator

Apparatus
  Simple
  Not expensive

---

was found between clinical findings and thermographic results, when the examination was carried out in the most serious cases of inflammatory disease of the joints. On the other hand, when the examination is conducted on joints with clinical signs of acute inflammation, but with less advanced disease, the results of thermography are positive in only 75% of the joints considered. So the first limitation of this method is the false negative results, especially in cases of deep and limited inflammation of the major joint.

But there are other disadvantages: the large superficial vessels, phlebo-thrombosis and some other vasculopathies, may cause false positive tests; the test is not specific in the sense that it evaluates any warm area, regardless of the etiology and the type of disease; the study is only quantitative; the machines are very expensive. However, the diffusion of thermographic techniques has been limited more by the high cost of the machines than by the other disadvantages.

At the moment it is possible to perform a good thermographic investigation using liquid crystals, which are not particularly expensive (Ambanelli et al., 1974b). The liquid crystals used are microcapsulated and have a range particularly suitable for human studies (temperatures between 32° and 36°C or between 36° and 40°C) (Di Roberto and Maggi, 1970). Liquid crystals may be directly applied over the cutaneous surface or, better, first placed over a resin and then applied over the joints for which the examination is requested. The hyperthermic areas appear colored in a way strictly related to the temperature present over the diseased joint and to the thermic fluctuation of the crystals applied. Usually, the modification of the colour goes from black in the colder areas to red in the areas at least 1°C warmer, to green in areas 2°C warmer, and finally to blue in areas which are 3°C or more warmer than the basal values.

We think that the application of the crystals over the resin gives better results in routine rheumatologic investigations, although we also had good results with the other technique. With plates, the investigation is much easier to perform; may be repeated shortly; and may be performed even in areas with cutaneous lesions. It is not necessary to use any ink, which can only be removed from the cutaneous surface with some difficulty, thus precluding any further examination in a short period of time and the picture appears without any intermediate time, which is necessary to prepare and to spout the black ground and then the liquid crystals.

However, it may be difficult to get perfect adhesion between the resin plate and the articular surface, even using plates with flexible resins. This inconvenience may be present especially in the little joints of the hand and in all cases with the most serious pathological lesions. In these cases it is much better to perform the thermographic study by liquid crystals directly applied over the articular surface, because the absence of adherence between the plate and the skin may give false negative results.

In inflammatory diseases of the joints, thermographic studies performed with liquid crystals give results comparable to those obtained by telethermographic investigations. The effectiveness of therapy may also be studied (Ambanelli, 1975). However, even this technique has disadvantages, e.g. false negative responses in 25% of cases, aspecificity, false positive responses due to inflammatory angiopathies, and the impossibility of obtaining a quantitative evaluation.

In conclusion, objective evaluation of local heat, whatever the method of registration, can give a good evaluation of the pathologic process at the articular level; however, it should be stressed that each method has its own inconveniences, and that only major differences between pre- and post-therapeutic findings should be considered really significant.

We have underlined that thermography gives only qualitative data. However, Collins et al. (1974) have recently reported some methods of quantitative study. They developed a thermographic index, i.e. the difference between the temperature found over inflamed joints and the temperature registered over the same joints in a group of normal healthy controls. However, the evaluation of the anti-inflammatory activity of any pharmacological agent requires strict standardization of methods, reduction of the percentage of false positive and false negative tests, and, above all, that the surface explored is always the same. But it is not easy and not always possible to work in standard conditions, which would reduce the number of faulty examinations.

To calculate the thermographic index, various areas of 10 cm^2 are chosen, for instance over the knee joint. These areas may be smaller in other joints, since the temperatures are referred to the unit of surface. After proper anti-inflammatory therapy, the thermographic index has been found to change in the case of rheumatoid arthritis, but it should be underlined that this technique is not easy and requires experience and skill in this particular field. This is one of the reasons why thermography is not at the moment a routine investigation.

A quantitative adaptation may be applied to thermographic machines, but not to all the other methods of thermographic investigation. We tried a quantitative investigation using liquid crystals. The theoretic basis is the same as described above. The colors, i.e. the temperatures, were read by photoelectric cells, examining circumscribed warm areas or previously defining the areas in comparison far from the warm areas. The results achieved are certainly interesting, but this method is not yet recommendable for routine application or for evaluation of the inflammatory activity of pharmacological agents.

Isotopic techniques can be used to make a quantitative investigation of articular inflammation. The isotopes used in rheumatologic studies have a short half-life, do not harm the patient, and quickly and electively become localized in the inflamed joints.

These methods are quite complicated and have been introduced only recently, even if much has been reported on this field in the world literature (Ahlstrom et al., 1956; Weiss et al., 1965; Glickmann et al., 1970; Dick et al., 1970a,b; Oka et al., 1970, 1973; Maxfield and Weiss, 1969; McCarty et al., 1970a,b; Sholkoff and Glickmann, 1969; Sholkoff et al., 1969; Whaley et al., 1968; Delbarre et al., 1971; St. Onge et al., 1968; Ambanelli and Ugolotti, 1971, 1972; Ambanelli et al., 1973, 1975; Huskisson et al., 1973).

It is now well known that these techniques clearly show the warm areas, corresponding to the joints clinically involved by the disease, even in the case of little joints or joints with circumscribed inflammation (Ambanelli et al., 1973). However, these techniques, even if interesting and useful, have their limits. especially as regards: aspecificity; impossibility of studying all the joints; difficulty of achieving quantitative data. Thus they are far from ideal. Perhaps, isotopic methods, applied as described above, are most useful for semiquantitative evaluation.

However, the machines we have in our laboratories may be used for a quantitative study by following a strict standard method of investigation and suppressing the great number of factors which may influence the system, such as dose, distance of the joint studied, surface of the joint studied, etc. Complying with some of these factors, Dick et al. (1970a,b) were able to calculate the percentage of isotope uptake by some inflamed joints. Other research workers in this field avoided the 'dose factor' and made all the investigations in comparison.

Following these criteria, we have been able to study a quantitative isotopic technique in which the key value is the ratio between the uptake found over the inflamed joint and that found over a muscular-cutaneous segment chosen as healthy control (Ambanelli and Ugolotti, 1972; Ambanelli et al., 1973). This same method has also been followed by Japanese workers and it does not differ significantly from that proposed by Oka et al. (1973), although their technique is based on different control values, such as uptake of bladder and heart. In the case of active inflammatory joint disease, this ratio has been found to be remarkably higher than in controls.

The sum of the values obtained in the eight joints considered for the investigation has been taken as the General Index of Inflammation; this has been called the Index of Articular Uptake, i.e. an index of evaluation of the disease as an entity. This index is: (1) higher in cases of rheumatoid arthritis; (2) related to some index of inflammation; and (3) enables one to follow the clinical history of the disease in parallel with other parameters (Ambanelli et al., 1973).

We report here the results of our experiments, but similar results were achieved by others (Oka et al., 1973) following similar techniques based on isotope uptake. However, these methods, even if applied successfully in clinical experience, should not be considered perfect or definitive. In fact, technical improvements have been suggested recently (such as collimator) and we think that these techniques will be greatly improved with the application of computers.

However, we think that all the quantitative techniques using technetium should be accepted with caution. The picture of an inflamed joint obtained using this isotope (which is the most used for qualitative investigations) is related to the vascularization, but also to the proteic linkage of the isotope (Green and Hays, 1969), which is particularly strong and which may be modified by the different concentrations of some anti-inflammatory agents (Ambanelli et al., 1974c).

It may thus be concluded that the isotopic pictures given by technetium are particularly helpful to the rheumatologist as regards diagnostic information on inflammation and grade of articular involvement, but for the study of the anti-inflammatory properties of a pharmacological agent it is better to use isotopes which (1) show only the vascular phase; (2) have no proteic linkage to be modified by the drugs considered; (3) have no problem of recirculation. An alternative technique might be thermographic investigation, which is sometimes preferable for study of the anti-inflammatory properties of an agent.

We underlined that the proteic linkage of the isotope is very strong and that it may be significantly influenced by some anti-inflammatory agents. On the other hand, thermographic investigation is strictly dependent on the cutaneous temperature and the grade of hyperemia so that, if the drug taken into consideration has no activity over the vessels, any modification of the thermogra-

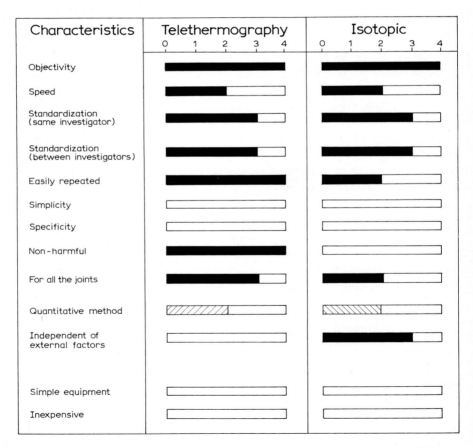

Fig. 1. Comparison of characteristics and validity (on an arbitrary scale of 0–4) of telethermography and isotopic methods.

TABLE 2

Comparison between thermography using liquid crystals and isotopic methods

Characteristics	Thermography by liquid crystals	Isotopic methods
Objectivity	present	present
Danger	none	depends on the isotope used
Evaluation of a fundamental symptom	hyperthermia	chiefly hyperthermia
Equipment	inexpensive	expensive
Qualified personnel	not required	required
Time involved for patient and investigator	brief	protracted
May be repeated	easily	not immediately
Casual errors	easily made: temperature change; cutaneous lesions, etc.	more difficult: technical pitfalls
Nonspecific evaluation of inflammation	present	present
Quantitative study	very difficult	possible
Localization of the inflamed area	moderate	very good

phic picture is related to the capability of the drug to act on articular inflammation.

At this point, before evaluating the other signs of inflammation, we think it advisable to make a comparison between the advantages and disadvantages of the different methods considered so far (Fig. 1), so it will be possible to draw some conclusions. The scale is arbitrary, but corresponds to growing degrees of validity of the method. For instance, it may be seen that the objectivity is high for both methods, the duration of the investigation is relatively short, the diagnostic possibilities good, etc. Finally, in Table 2 isotopes and liquid crystals are compared.

The tumefaction of the joints may be easily evaluated by simple machines (artrometers) or by radiologic investigations. To obtain information on the soft tissues, even in the case of light or initial involvement, it is necessary to observe some technical points (thin focus, films of particular sensitiveness, accurate manual processing), which are certainly well known to all radiologists, but require remarkable care. So in routine practice it is not always possible to have good results. However, all the morphologic disorders, both initial and late, of inflammatory joint disease, may now be studied by *xerography*, a technique which is even better than the traditional radiologic investigations.

The data derived from radiological study are extremely important from a diagnostic point of view, but less useful as regards the evaluation of any change which follows short-term anti-inflammatory therapy. Moreover, joint size is not always directly proportional to the seriousness of the inflammatory disease. We have no other technical method which allows an evaluation of the other signs of inflammation which could be more significant than that given by clinical examination. Here we will only comment briefly on some new techniques which have been recently reported. Since we have some experience with them, we report here some conclusions from the results we achieved.

According to Vadasz (1971) strain-gauge plethysmography could be useful for evaluating the anti-inflammatory properties of pharmacological agents. We found some differences between the pre- and post-therapy pictures, but they were not constant and so we do not think that Vadasz's method should be recommended for routine evaluation of drugs.

Other research workers tried to give an objective evaluation of articular stiffness (Wright and Johns, 1960; Ingpen and Kendall, 1968; Hicklin et al., 1968; Backlund and Tiselius, 1967; Ambanelli et al., 1974a). The most interesting methods are those which evoke a passive movement of the joint and then record resistances. Our own technique follows this theoretic basis, but it explores only one joint, so we will not report here any details concerning the results (Ambanelli and Giannini, 1973).

We recorded some graphic representations which are quite different in cases of rheumatoid arthritis than in normal healthy controls. The pictures recorded in cases of rheumatoid arthritis are completely different, depending on the presence or absence of and the degree of inflammation. We would emphasize that the only joint which may be explored by this technique is the metacarpophalangeal. The instrumental recording of joint stiffness gives interesting graphic representations, but requires a high degree of technical sophistication to reduce the numerous parameters which, even in this method, influence the results. Otherwise, it will not be possible to make any comparisons.

Excluding the large number of technical problems reported elsewhere (Ambanelli et al., 1973, 1975), which in our opinion limit the applicability of this technique, we think that the most important restriction is that only the stiffness of the metacarpophalangeal joint of the second finger can be investigated. Moreover, the joint must not have anatomical damage so serious as to limit its own movements. In other words, this technique studies only patients affected by rheumatoid arthritis with involvement of the metacarpophalangeal joints, with a brief clinical history and without relevant morphological lesions. In conclusion, the method is not suitable for the greater number of patients affected by rheumatoid arthritis or for routine investigations.

We have not considered methods such as arthroscopy, which is useful for diagnosis but not for the evaluation of the anti-inflammatory properties of non-steroid agents, but we conclude that none of the instrumental methods proposed so far can be considered as ideal for studying a diseased joint. In fact, all the instrumental methods, even if apparently accurate, have an inherent percentage of false positive and false negative results and a certain number of disadvantages. Moreover, the techniques discussed, even those most used (such as thermography and isotopic methods), require complex and expensive equipment, which limits their routine application in clinical practice.

However, we do not want to give an impression of absolutely negative conclusions or of exaggerated pessimism. We only wish to stress that, even using the most sophisticated and modern techniques, it is particularly difficult to evaluate the therapeutic properties of an anti-inflammatory agent. Methods are still imperfect, but the progress of the last few years should stimulate rheumatologists to go on with the instrumental evaluation of joint inflammation.

References

AHLSTROM, S., GEDDA, P. O. and HEDBERG, H. (1956): Disappearance of radioactive serum albumin from joints in rheumatoid arthritis. *Acta rheum. scand.*, 2, 219.

AMBANELLI, U. (1975): Valutazione preliminare di alcuni indici di flogosi. La termografia. In: *Atti, VI Congresso S.S.F.A., Tirrenia, 20–21 June 1975.*

AMBANELLI, U. and GIANNINI, A. (1973): Considerazioni su di una metodica quantitativa della rigidità articolare. In: *Atti, Congresso, Sez. Tosco-Umbro-Emiliana, Società Italiana di Reumatologia, Montecatini Terme, 7 April 1973.*

AMBANELLI, U., GIANNINI, A. and MANGANELLI, P. (1974a): Tentativo di valutazione obiettiva della rigidità articolare nell'artrite reumatoide. *Reumatismo*, 26, 780.

AMBANELLI, U., NERVETTI, A. and DI ROBERTO, F. (1974b): L'impiego della termografia con cristalli liquidi nella diagnostica delle reumopatie flogistiche. In: *Atti, XXI Congresso della Società Italiana di Reumatologia, Montecatini Terme, 8–10 November 1974.*

AMBANELLI, U., NERVETTI, A. and UGOLOTTI, G. (1974c): Valutazione comparata della flogosi articolare. Confronto tra le immagini scintigrafiche ed i rilievi termografici. In: *Atti, XXI Congresso delia Società Italiana di Reumatologia, Montecatini Terme, 8–10 November 1974.*

AMBANELLI, U. and UGOLOTTI, G. (1971): Szintifotografische Beurteilung der Gelenkentzündung. *Arzneimittel-Forsch.*, 21, 802.

AMBANELLI, U. and UGOLOTTI, G. (1972): Valore e limiti delle indagini scintigrafiche e scintifotografiche nell'artrite reumatoide. In: *Atti, XXV Congresso Nazionale di Radiologia Medica e di Medicina Nucleare, Montecatini, 1–4 June 1972.*

AMBANELLI, U., UGOLOTTI, G., NERVETTI, A. and MANGANELLI, P. (1975): L'emploi des nouveaux isotopes ostéotropes dans les maladies ostéo-articulaires, avec attention particulière pour les arthropathies phlogistiques. *Rev. Rhum.*, 42, 513.

AMBANELLI, U., UGOLOTTI, G., NERVETTI, A. and TROISE, W. (1973): Evaluation isotopique quantitative de la phlogose articulaire. *Rev. Rhum.*, 40, 419.

BACKLUND, L. and TISELIUS, P. (1967): Objective measurement of joint stiffness in rheumatoid arthritis. *Acta rheum. scand.*, 13, 275.

COLLINS, A. J., RING, E. F. J., COSH, J. A. and BACON, P. A. (1974): Quantitation of thermography in arthritis using multi-isothermal analysis. I. The thermographic index. *Ann. rheum. Dis.*, *33*, 113.

COSH, J. A. and RING, E. F. J. (1970): Thermography and rheumatology. *Rheumatol. Phys. Med.*, *10*, 342.

DELBARRE, F., ROUCAYROL, J. C., MENKES, C. I., PRIN, P., INGRAND, J., REBUT, C. and AIGNAN, M. (1971): Intérêt de l'arthroscintigraphie au technétium-^{99m}Tc, par voie intraveineuse dans l'étude des processus inflammatoires. *Rev. Rhum.*, *38*, 91.

DICK, W. C., NEUFELD, R. R., PRENTICE, A. G., WOODBURN, A., WHALEY, K., NUKI, G. and BUCHANAN, W. W. (1970a): Measurement of joint inflammation: a radioisotopic method. *Ann. rheum. Dis.*, *29*, 135.

DICK, W. C., WHALEY, K., ST. ONGE, R. A., DOWNIE, W. W., BOYLE, J. A., NUKI, G., GILLESPIE, F. C. and BUCHANAN, W. W. (1970b): Clinical studies on inflammation in human knee joints: xenon (^{133}Xe) clearances correlated with clinical assessment in various arthritides and studies on the effect of intra-articularly administered hydrocortisone in rheumatoid arthritis. *Clin. Sci.*, *38*, 123.

DI ROBERTO, F. and MAGGI, G. C. (1970): La termografia cutanea a cristalli liquidi microincapsulati. *Bassini*, *15*, 3.

GLICKMAN, M. G., SHOLKOFF, S. D. and GILBERT, R. J. (1970): Appearance of normal peripheral joints by scintiphotography. *Invest. Radiol.*, *5*, 50.

GREEN, F. A. and HAYS, M. T. (1969): Joint scanning: mechanism and application. *Arthr. and Rheum.*, *12*, 299.

HABERMAN, J. A., SISK, C. W., TOURTELLOTTE, C. D., BIRTWELL, W. M. and MARTIN, J. H. (1971): Thermography in arthritis. *Arthr. and Rheum.*, *14*, 387.

HICKLIN, J., WIGHTON, R. J. and ROBINSON, F. J. (1968): Measurement of finger stiffness. *Ann. phys. Med.*, *9*, 234.

HUSKISSON, E. C. (1974): La misura della malattia. In: *Atti, Simposio Internazionale sulla Reumatologia*. Fondazione Carlo Erba, Milan.

HUSKISSON, E. C., BERRY, H., BROWETT, J. P. and BALME, H. W. (1973): Comparison of technetium clearance and thermography with standard methods in a clinical trial. *Ann. rheum. Dis.*, *32*, 99.

INGPEN, P. L. and KENDALL, P. H. (1968): A simple apparatus for assessment of stiffness. *Ann. phys. Med.*, *9*, 203.

MAXFIELD, W. S. and WEISS, T. T. (1969): Technetium-99m joint images. *Radiology*, *92*, 1461.

McCARTY, D. J., POLCYN, R. E. and COLLINS, P. A. (1970a): 99m-Technetium scintiphotography in arthritis. II. Its nonspecificity and clinical and roentgenographic correlations in rheumatoid arthritis. *Arthr. and Rheum.*, *13*, 21.

McCARTY, D. J., POLCYN, R. E., COLLINS, P. A. and GOTTSCHALK, A. (1970b): Technetium scintiphotography in arthritis. I. Technic and interpretation. *Arthr. and Rheum.*, *13*, 11.

OKA, M., REKONEN, A. and ROUTSI, A. (1970): Technetium-99m in the study of rheumatic joints. *Acta rheum. scand.*, *16*, 271.

OKA, M., REKONEN, A., ROUTSI, A. and KNIKKA, J. (1973): Measurement of systemic inflammatory activity in rheumatoid arthritis by the ^{99m}Tc method. *Scand. J. Rheumatol.*, *2*, 101.

PASERO, G. (1975): Problemi metodologici relativi alla valutazione clinica dei farmaci antiflogistici nell'artrite reumatoide. In: *Atti, Simposio Internazionale sulla Reumatologia, S. Margherita di Pula, 18–20 April 1975.*

RING, E. F. J. and COLLINS, A. J. (1970): Quantitative thermography. *Rheumatol. phys. Med.,* *10,* 337.

RING, E. F. J., COLLINS, A. J., BACON, P. A. and COSH, J. A. (1974): Quantitation of thermography in arthritis using multi-isothermal analysis. II. Effect of non-steroidal anti-inflammatory therapy on the thermographic index. *Ann. rheum. Dis.,* *33,* 353.

SHOLKOFF, S. D. and GLICKMAN, M. G. (1969): Scintiphotographic evaluation of arthritis activity. *Invest. Radiol.,* *4,* 207.

SHOLKOFF, S. D., GLICKMAN, M. G., SHACHTER, J. and ROWLAND, M. (1969): External counting and scintiphotography in rabbits with arthritis. *Arthr. and Rheum.,* *12,* 220.

ST. ONGE, R. A., DICK, W. C., BELL, G. and BOYLE, J. A. (1968): Radioactive xenon (^{133}Xe) disappearance rates from the synovial cavity of the human knee joint in normal and arthritis subjects. *Ann. rheum. Dis.,* *27,* 163.

VADASZ, I. (1971): Straingauge plethysmography in the assessment of joint inflammation. *Ann. rheum. Dis.,* *30,* 194.

WEISS, T. E., MAXFIELD, W. S., MURISON, P. J. and HIDALGO, J. U. (1965): Iodinated human serum albumin (I^{131}) localization studies of rheumatoid arthritis joints by scintillation scanning. *Arthr. and Rheum.,* *8,* 976.

WHALEY, K., PACK, A. I., BOYLE, J. A., DICK, W. C., DOWNIE, W. W., BUCHANAN, W. W. and GILLESPIE, F. C. (1968): The articular scan in rheumatoid arthritis: a possible method of quantitating joint inflammation using radio-technetium. *Clin. Sci.,* *35,* 547.

WRIGHT, V. and JOHNS, R. J. (1960): Observations on the measurement of joint stiffness. *Arthr. and Rheum.,* *3,* 328.

Chrysotherapy: its value and means of action

F. Buneaux, J.-J. Buneaux, P. Fabiani and P. Galmiche

Laboratoire Central de Biochimie, Hôtel-Dieu, Paris and Hôpital de Neuilly, France

It was in 1929 that J. Forestier first introduced gold salts for the treatment of rheumatism. Gold salts are consequently one of our oldest important medications, even if the idea upon which their application was based, was subsequently shown to be incorrect (an analogy with tuberculosis, which was commonly treated with gold salts). We still do not know a great deal about the mechanism of action of the treatment, which has received little interest, largely on account of the side effects which its use can induce. Yet these side effects are neither more serious nor more frequent than those to which many patients are subjected under other modern therapies, which are nonetheless widely used (corticoids, immuno-suppressors, D-penicillamine and numerous anti-inflammatory agents). In order to give a reasonable overview of chrysotherapy, we would like to stress two points: side effects and the mechanism of action.

The statistical comparison of the frequency and gravity of the side effects with the value and duration of successful treatment has demonstrated that the use of chrysotherapy deserves not only to be continued, but to be praised. On the occasion of the recent Round Table presided over by Mme V. May, Renier, Louyot and other members of the *Société Française de Rhumatologie* underlined these points (*Rev. Rhum.*, 1971, *38 (II)*, 669). In this article we will do no more than refer to their conclusions, since further statistics cannot add a great deal to what seems to be proven. Instead we shall give a personal opinion. We have been impressed by the accomplishment of some American authors, who have also attempted to elucidate these two problems.

Side effects

The clinical side effects of chrysotherapy are very diverse: mucocutaneous, digestive, renal, and, more rarely, jaundice, bronchitis, or polyneuritis. It does not seem necessary to consider the toxicity of gold by thesaurismosis, since some patients were subjected to large and repeated doses without the slightest incident. The general consensus is that it is a question of hypersensitivity in which the complex of a serum protein and gold salts acts as an antigen.

This sensitisation can be detected by laboratory tests, which, however, are not yet widely practised: Denmann's lymphoblastic transformation test; Shelley's mastocytary degradation test; and Louyot's leukocyte migration inhibition test. Thus it should be possible to distinguish between hereditary and acquired sensitisation and to distinguish the real cause of any accident or side effect during the course of treatment. Nonetheless, a wider application of these difficult tests seems to us to be necessary before their specificity can be confirmed.

The levels of gold in the blood, urine and the pathological fluids can be measured, first by colorimetric methods (Block and Buchanan, 1940), as used by Freyberg et al. (1972), and then, very precisely and reliably, by the atomic absorption method (Lorber et al., 1973). These measurements have enabled a variety of investigations to be carried out.

Researchers have attempted to determine the level of chrysemy necessary, and to achieve its maintenance, in order to be able to prolong the action of the treatment and guarantee its success. This hope has proved to be vain, because there is no optimum chrysemy, any more than there is a threshold dose of toxicity. Certain subjects experienced very good results with only small doses. French authors do not consider that this technique presents any great advantages over Forestier's traditional technique. It is to this technique, perhaps for reasons of routine and ease, that we returned. In any case, Rothermich et al. (1967) have shown that the results do not depend on the dose.*
Furthermore, this technique offers no escape from side effects. In our opinion, the necessary therapeutic dose is very close to an overdose, but this varies from patient to patient.

Lewis and Ziff (1966) have recommended and experimented with intra-articular injection of gold salts. But the gold is not fixed on the synovial membrane to any extent, at least we did not detect any more than with other

---

*Those dosages are not simple. Among other problems, they have to be administered at a precise moment in relation to the last injection of gold salts, and this is not always straight-forward in the case of outpatients.

methods. It remains only a short while in the synovial fluid, and the results of this technique, which is more complicated than intra-muscular injection, are no better.

The frequency of side effects has been exaggerated because of their potential seriousness, and this has given many people the false impression that chrysotherapy is dangerous, whereas in fact it just needs care. The side effects are seen particularly in badly conducted treatments. In our opinion, chrysotherapy should be used alone, with no adjuvants. Such adjuvants serve only to disguise the first signs of intolerance, without avoiding them. Therapy should be terminated at the first such sign, unless, perhaps, the tests of which we have spoken indicate that the gold is not responsible.

These side effects are henceforth entirely capable of therapeutic correction. We would simply mention that since the use of BAL (dimercaprol), good results have been obtained from other chelates (EDTA, D-penicillamine) and cortisone. We have not had the opportunity of trying N-acetyl-cysteine, which, in the opinion of Lorber et al. (1973), is similarly extremely active.

In conclusion, we suggest that the side effects of gold are rare in a well conducted treatment, and that, thanks to the new possibility of treatment of these side effects, they no longer present serious problems. This of course does not imply the institution of chrysotherapy for rheumatoid arthritis without adequate trials, but, on the other hand, it would be a mistake to systematically ignore an effective therapy.

Mechanism of action

The effectiveness of gold in the treatment of rheumatoid arthritis is equally difficult to explain. How and why does it work? It is one thing to point out its therapeutic benefits, but the explanation and understanding of these benefits is far more difficult. Thus, in animals, gold prevents experimental arthritis due to arthriditic mycoplasma, but not that due to Freund's adjuvant (where, nonetheless, it has a certain effect.) For several years there has been a general orientation towards the idea that gold causes an inactivation of an enzyme system. Weissmann (1966) was one of the first to draw attention to this point.

In vitro ionised gold inhibits the capacity of trypsic inhibition (Buneaux et al., 1975a). Gottlieb et al. (1975) think that the gold may block an alpha-2-macroglobulin, the absence of which permits the erosion of the hyaline cartilage by proteolytic enzymes. But the proteins which are the site of the anti-protease activity (the main one being the alpha-1-antitrypsin) do not seem to be modified in rheumatic arthritis (Buneaux et al., 1975b).

Gold also inhibits other enzyme activities such as β-glucuronidase, cytofibrokinase and malate dehydrogenase. In our research we tried to discover whether gold was an inactivator of the synovial enzymes, the concentrations of which we found to be higher in the synovial fluids of patients suffering from this disease (Buneaux et al., 1975b). Thus, from research in vitro and on normal human serum, we have found that LDH is inhibited by 14% when 100 μg/ml of Au^{+++} are added; for 150 μg/ml the diminution is 22% and for 200 μg/ml, it is 32%. Lysozyme is only 5% inactivated for 100 μg/ml, 18% for 150 μg/ml, and 28% for 200 μg/ml. Acid phosphatase is the most sensitive. It is inhibited, although only partially, for concentrations as weak as 2.5 μg/ml.

These three lysosomal enzymes were found to be greatly increased in the inflammatory articular fluids of rheumatoid arthritis cases, just as was betaglucuronidase, but, for this last enzyme, lysosomal also, gold proved to be inactive at concentrations of 200 μg/ml. Furthermore, gold is also inactive in inhibiting enzymes, the concentration of which we did not find to be increased in cases of rheumatoid arthritis: SGOT, SGPT, alkaline phosphatase and amylase.

Gold alone seems to have these properties. Metals with an atomic weight close to that of gold (thallium, mercury, lead) do not give the same inhibitory effects. Only platinum, gold's neighbour on Mendeleeff's table, behaves like gold on the capacity of trypsic inhibition.

There is thus a strong temptation to point to this as the therapeutic mode of action. But the mode of action of gold which we identified in vitro requires strong concentrations, larger than those used in therapy. For this reason, after having confirmed with an isotopic scintigraph that in animals the gold is concentrated at the level of the hepato-nephro-splenic reticuloendothelial system (Buneaux et al., 1973), by whatever means it is introduced, we concluded that it was there that the therapeutic action of the gold was exercised, since it is also at this level that the antibodies are formed. But there is a difficulty, namely that the serum enzymes are not found to be decreased in number, or diminished in effectiveness. How then can we explain the articular improvement?

In animal studies the gold is not concentrated at the level of the arthritic membrane provoked by carragheenin, nor at the level of the hypophysis (Buneaux et al., 1973). Rather, as we have pointed out, it is concentrated at the level of the splanchnic viscera.

In man, we have seen that gold does not remain for long in the synovial fluid, that it traverses the membrane without becoming fixed to it, and that it does not alter the number of serum enzymes. How, then, are we to understand its action from an enzymatic point of view? It is difficult. Nevertheless, it is certain that all the enzymes, the concentration of which we have measured in the synovial fluid, are the ones which pass through it, and which remain there a short time. What we measure is nothing but a moment in the perpetual interaction between enzymes and anti-enzymes.

So, to conclude, it now seems to us that, if gold acts enzymatically, it is at the level of the cells themselves, of the lysosomes, and that its action must be detected, perhaps when the gold is in its ionic form Au^{+++}, and in weak concentration. The inhibited enzymes are above all lysosomal, even though some of them remain unaffected. Only through intracellular microchemical research can this hypothesis be confirmed or invalidated. But the hypothesis certainly makes it worthwhile for the research of Weissmann (1966) to be taken up again, pursued and clarified.

Conclusions

Without belittling the achievements of modern therapies for rheumatoid arthritis (immuno-suppressors, D-penicillamine), we can say that their brilliant results do not make the use of chrysotherapy worthless. Chrysotherapy can provide unquestionable, frequent and lasting successes, which it would be wrong to ignore. The therapeutic indication for chrysotherapy remains an early indication, particularly in the case of a young sufferer, and when the diagnosis is certain, that is to say when all the criteria of rheumatoid arthritis are present.

Thus we maintain that this old medical treatment is still valuable, and warrants continued application. Even if at present we are unable to fully master the inconveniences it presents, and even if we do not yet fully understand its mode of action, modern research is suggesting a new orientation for its application, which may one day lead to the solution of the problem.

References

BLOCK, W. D. and BUCHANAN, O. H. (1940): The microdetermination of gold in biological fluids. *J. biol. Chem.*, *136*, 379.

BUNEAUX, F., LUCROQ, M. B. and GALMICHE, P. (1973): Recherches sur le chrysothérapie. *Rev. Rhum.*, *40 (6)*, 429.

BUNEAUX, J.-J., BUNEAUX, F. and GALMICHE, P. (1975a): Action de l'ion Au $^{+++}$ sur la capacité d'inhibition trypsique et élastasique du sérum. *INSERM. 40*, 141.

BUNEAUX, J.-J., BUNEAUX, F. and GALMICHE, P. (1975b): Quelques enzymes synoviales dans la polyarthrite rhumatoïde. *Rev. Rhum.*, *42 (2)*, 97.

FORESTIER, J. (1971): Traitement de la polyarthrite chronique évolutive par le chrysothérapie. *Rev. Rhum.*, *38 (II)*, 669.

FREYBERG, R. H., ZIFF, M. and BAYM, J. (1972): In: *Gold Therapy for Rheumatoid Arthritis, Arthritis and Allied Conditions*, p. 455. Editors: J. L. Hollander and D. J. McCarty. Lea and Febiger, Philadelphia.

GOTTLIEB, N. L., KIEM, I. M., PENNEYS, N. S. and SCHULTZ, D. R. (1975): The influence of chrysotherapy on serum protein and immunoglobulin levels, rheumatoid factor and anti-epithelial antibody titers. *J. Lab. clin. Med.*, *86*, 962.

LEWIS, D. C. and ZIFF, M. (1966): Intra-articular administration of gold salts. *Arthr. and Rheum.*, *9*, 682.

LORBER, A. ATKINS, C. J., CHANG, C. C., LEE, Y. B., STARS, J. and BOVY, R. A. (1973): Monitoring serum gold values to improve chrysotherapy in R.A. *Ann. rheum. Dis.*, *32*, 133.

ROTHERMICH, N. O., BERGEN, W. and PHILIPS, V. K. (1967): The use of plasma gold levels in determining dose frequency, type of gold salts and impending toxicity in chrysotherapy for R.A. *Arthr. and Rheum.*, *10*, 308.

WEISSMANN, G. (1966): Lysosomes and joint diseases. *Arthr. and Rheum.*, *9*, 834.

IIIA. *Past, present and future of indomethacin*

Chairman D. P. Barcelo
Co-chairman D. Gigante

Introduction

D. Gigante

Istituto di Reumatologia, University of Rome, Italy

The purpose of the present session is to analyse the abundance of data gathered on indomethacin in years of intensive work, to point out the benefits this medicament can bring as well as the limitations imposed by its side effects, and to envisage, in the light of the information acquired so far, what will be its future role in the therapy of rheumatic diseases.

There has been an exhaustive discussion, also in the framework of the present Symposium, as to the evaluation of the activity of anti-inflammatory drugs, the different criteria to be applied for the various diseases, and the possible methods of experimentation.

All of this seems to be indispensable for each and every preparation before it receives official recognition and judgement and is put on the test-bench of free prescription by doctors, spontaneous acceptance by patients and competition with other drugs. Under such conditions many a medicament has proved to be of little value and failed to stand the test of time, whereas only a few have become established and made further progress.

This is the case with indomethacin, synthetised in the 1960s in the West Point research laboratories of Merck, Sharp and Dohme and now marketed in over 170 countries throughout the world. It has been the object of very thorough studies reported in over two thousand publications and has been discussed in detail in recent Congresses on Rheumatology, so much so that no further illustration is needed.

I will therefore confine myself to just a few introductory remarks and to outlining a few problems. I am also convinced that a deeper knowledge of the properties of indomethacin–which at present can be considered as the model of anti-inflammatory non-steroidal drugs–will also contribute to the definition of other medicaments of the same type.

Anti-inflammatory activity, general and at the same time selective for certain processes of morbidity, is peculiar to only a few, very active drugs, such as phenylbutazone and indomethacin. How and why such a discriminating property comes into action is still an open question: it is possible to assume that the varying efficacy shown by indomethacin in different diseases depends on the type of inflammation characterizing the disease and on the different structures involved. One example is the widely differing effects which may be obtained in ankylosing spondylitis and rheumatoid arthritis.

Indomethacin yields better results in ankylosing spondylitis when it is confined to the spine. On the other hand, the beneficial effects of its administration are reduced, very much the same as observed in rheumatoid arthritis, when there is involvement of peripheral joints in ankylosing spondylitis.

In acute gouty attack, where a model of microcrystalline arthritis may be spotted and reappears with the same characteristics in subsequent episodes, the anti-inflammatory activity of indomethacin is paradigmatic and repeatable. Less evident and constant effects are obtained in uratic arthritis when the phlogistic process becomes chronic and gout presents tophaceous aspects.

Although it may be argued that individual sensitivity to indomethacin varies, it is my opinion that the differences observed between individual patients with the same disease can be attributed to the severity, magnitude and stage of advancement of the pathological process, to the regions involved, and to other conditions inherent in the individual case which often baffle even a careful investigator. This might account for the discrepancies in results achieved with the same dose schedules in groups of patients selected according to homogeneous criteria.

It is quite easily understandable, for instance, that in rheumatoid arthritis more evident effects are obtained in the early stages and in oligo-articular cases, when there is an acute febrile onset or a more intense inflammatory activity, and when there is no previous record of cortisone drug administration.

In this connection another interesting example is provided by degenerative arthropathies, where the efficacy of indomethacin seems to vary depending on whether osteoarthritis is primary or secondary in character, according to the location, severity and stage of development of the diseases. This is clearly demonstrated by osteoarthritis of the hip, where indomethacin proves extremely active, so that it is the medicament of choice. And yet, the results range from good to excellent in about two-thirds of cases, but are modest or absent in the remaining cases. In order to account for this discrepancy, I think it necessary to go back to the origin of pain, which in osteoarthritis of the hip depends on different factors that prevail in turn in the individual cases, so that three major groups may be outlined.

In the first group, the origin of pain is related to structural arthritic alterations and basically lies in the periosteum and the subchondral bone. Pain is therefore provoked by movement of the joints, especially under load, and disappears on rest. In my opinion, this is the group of cases where indomethacin scores good or moderate results (only rarely excellent results) and a share of failures. The effect, when it is present, is clearly of a temporary nature, since pain is quickly relieved but reappears after discontinuation of the drug therapy.

Long-term treatment will therefore be established, and the evening administration of a 100 mg suppository is quite appropriate. It has the advantage of allowing for some activity, such as housework, to be performed the following morning. This therapy basically maintains its efficacy over time, unless the arthritic lesions deteriorate sharply.

In the second group, pain has a basically mechanical origin and is due to stress, strain, compression and continued microtraumatism of the peri-articular soft tissues and consequently of the capsule of the joint when subjected to various movements. This syndrome may also imply modifications in the angle of inclination of the thigh bone and, in relation to a valgus neck, it may impose a static-functional overload on the upper lateral part of the femoral head, thus increasing the wear of cartilage at that level. All of this is a pre-condition for the development of anatomical incongruities in the centred forms of osteoarthritis of the hip and for deterioration of de-centred forms, notably those with upper polar involvement. In these cases indomethacin seems less useful, or inefficient altogether, since only its analgesic properties are utilised, whereas its main asset, the anti-inflammatory capacity, has no role to play.

Far better is the response to indomethacin in the third group of cases, where capsule-synovial or fibrotic inflammation of the peri-articular tissues superimposes on the degenerative process of the joints. The resulting hyperalgesic *poussée* persists at rest and benefits from anti-inflammatory therapy. Indomethacin provides excellent results in the large majority of such cases, bringing about a remission of the painful symptoms related to the inflammatory component.

As far as functional impairment, the other major symptom of osteoarthritis of the hip, is concerned, indomethacin may improve the situation to the extent that impairment results from pain and muscle contractures and phlogistic alterations in ligaments, tendons and capsule. Articular motor dynamics are frequently restored as pain subsides; this is evident in deambulation and recorded by measuring the intercondyloid and intermalleolar distance. This effect is obviously more conspicuous in the case of osteoarthritis of the hip with superimposing inflammation. In contrast, little or nothing can be expected from the use of indomethacin when impaired movements are due to anatomical alterations in connections of joint bone endings, or the typical lesions of osteoarthritis, or static alterations.

Analysis of individual cases did not reveal any significant differences between primary and secondary osteoarthritis of the hip as far as the response to indomethacin was concerned. There was, however, a slightly higher frequency of positive results in centred as against de-centred forms. All in all, however, these parameters are difficult to detect in the absence of any close relationship between the severity of the anatomical-radiological lesions and the therapeutic response. It is also common knowledge that pain is not always proportional to the intensity of alterations and that it may be absent when the latter take on considerable importance.

Broadly speaking, however, indomethacin is more effective in the early stages of osteoarthritis of the hip, and the results are less good in the advanced and severe stages of the disease. More satisfactory results are attained in monolateral forms, and after them in bilateral forms with pain predominant on only one side.

A clear, though less well known, indication for indomethacin is provided by connective rheumatism, where excellent results are often scored in joint involvement with systemic lupus, polymyositis, scleroderma and nodose panarteritis. No effect is detectable on the basic process and visceral involvement.

Extra-articular rheumatisms of a fibrositic character lend themselves to management with indomethacin, but the broad variety of morbid forms they cover and the psychosomatic component they often present make it rather difficult to draw up a scheme of the objectively attainable results.

A number of real, organic fibrositis cases may benefit considerably, up to complete recovery; it is the other way round in the psychosomatic forms, where a further aggravation when the patients are on anti-rheumatic drug therapy points to the marked predominance of the psychogenic component.

As regards periarthritis of the shoulder, the best results are obtained in acute forms in the early stage, or in any case when no articular block has occurred.

The usefulness of indomethacin is well established and thoroughly documented in cervical brachialgia and particularly in the acute phase of lumbago. The analgesic effect proves to be the most evident of all, whereas the physical and, even more so, the neurological symptoms give a less favourable response. Failures therefore are basically related to the most advanced, obstinate and recidivist forms of disease and to the cases with serious disc lesions and consequent extensive osteoarthritic processes.

The advisability of associated anti-inflammatory treatments has been discussed at length, and the drugs and morbid conditions possibly suited for application have also been explored. I am convinced that when cortisone drugs are required their dose schedule can be substantially reduced by the simultaneous administration of indomethacin. As for the advisability of associating indomethacin with other non-steroidal anti-inflammatory drugs, this should be considered and evaluated on an individual basis for each patient; the judgement is often personal and not suited to be codified.

Contraindications to indomethacin are widely known, thanks also to the detailed and exhaustive information provided by Merck, Sharp and Dohme, who have most carefully and correctly reported all possible side effects, including the rarest ones. My experience with indomethacin is that it is quite well tolerated, all things considered, the stomach being the most vulnerable area. Many paediatricians tend to advise against indomethacin in children. This is perhaps over-cautious, although the use of indomethacin in children needs to be limited.

In conclusion, it is always difficult to express a judgement as to the future of a medicament, but in the case of indomethacin it is safe to say that it has brilliant prospects. It certainly cannot lose ground, and will enhance and extend its reputation, unless a new drug is developed which has the same effectiveness and possibly better tolerance.

Pharmacological and early clinical investigations

Norman O. Rothermich

Ohio State University, Columbus Medical Center Research Foundation, Columbus, Ohio, U.S.A.

In order to provide a background and a perspective for this session on indomethacin, I shall review briefly the state of anti-rheumatic therapy prior to indomethacin and some of the biochemical and basic pharmacological events involved in bringing this drug to the clinical level. Prior to 1949, anti-rheumatic therapy was at a low ebb, and rheumatoid patients were advised 'to take aspirin and learn to live with it'. Although parenteral gold therapy had been and is now regarded as highly effective in rheumatoid arthritis, at *that* time it had fallen into disrepute because of overdosage with many serious and sometimes fatal side effects.

In 1949 Dr. Hench and his co-workers from the Mayo Clinic provided one of the most dramatic moments in medical history when they announced the discovery of cortisone and demonstrated, at an international congress of many hundreds of physicians, the near miraculous benefit of cortisone on severely diseased rheumatoid arthritis. That these hundreds of physicians would stand up and cheer at this demonstration was eloquent testimonial to the psychologic impact and drama of this great moment. Not long afterward, cortisone derivatives began to appear, most notably prednisone which concentrated anti-rheumatic potency and eliminated much of the very distressing sodium- and water-retaining properties of cortisone; with this, cortisone therapy became an integral part of treatment.

At about this same time, another potent anti-rheumatic drug appeared on the horizon in the form of phenylbutazone marketed as Butazolidine. Although its effects in rheumatoid arthritis were of limited value, it provided striking benefit in patients with spondylitis, gout, osteoarthritis and similar 'benign' rheumatic diseases. Its many and sometimes serious side effects did not become apparent for several years, but did lead to curtailment of its usefulness.

Still, the continued importance of salicylates as the first line of anti-rheumatic drug therapy emphasized the serious dearth of potently effective anti-rheumatic drugs. Physicians had become increasingly aware of long-term hazards of high-dose cortisone therapy as well as the side effects and limitations of Butazolidine, and they remained reluctant to employ chrysotherapy. There was widespread proliferation of many quack remedies of arthritis.

About 1960, the now famous biochemist Dr. T. Y. Shen put together several isolated facts: (1) the controversial role of 5-hydroxytryptamine as a possible anti-inflammatory mediator; (2) the availability of a collection of indole derivatives previously studied in the serotonin-antagonist program; and (3) the finding of markedly increased excretion of tryptophan metabolites in rheumatoid arthritics. His interest was thus stimulated in indole derivatives as potential anti-rheumatic agents. From this, indomethacin was born.

I would like to quote from a recent communication from Dr. Shen: 'In the field of medicinal chemistry, the successful demonstration of a laboratory approach to arthritis has stimulated many more researchers (including ourselves) to find newer agents of this type, hopefully, with some improvements. This is evident from the hundreds of patents on aryl acetic acids filed by laboratories worldwide in the past decade. Perhaps our collective effort would advance the continuous struggle against arthritis one more step. From the basic science point of view, indomethacin, as a potent inhibitor of prostaglandin synthetase with 10 years' human and animal experience, has become a valuable research tool in the elucidation of the physiological roles of prostaglandins. Prostaglandins are produced in microgram quantities daily and only have a transient existence in target tissues. The judicious use of indomethacin in many experimental systems has not only reflected the consequence of prostaglandin deprivation but may unravel new therapeutic possibilities. In this sense, indomethacin is not merely a means to an end but also possibly a key to a new era of biomedical research.'

Extensive animal testing for therapeutic efficacy and side effects was carried out under the direction of Dr. Charles Winter. In this, he applied the new approaches which he had developed to produce inflammation in animals. The resulting inflammation could be and was used as test material for quantitating anti-inflammatory effects of various drugs. Of course, the translation of work with such synthetically induced inflammation in animals to the spontaneously occurring and unique rheumatic inflammation in humans is not always easy and may not always be valid. Nevertheless, it apparently proved to be so in the case with indomethacin.

The first clinical trial of indomethacin was begun by me in a 35-year-old woman in November, 1961. Serendipitously, the patient selected was suffering from ankylosing spondylitis, which is probably the only disease that would respond to the comparatively small doses initially employed, namely, 5 mg t.i.d. and then 10 mg t.i.d. At the latter dose a definite clinical benefit was discernible. The good result in this trial encouraged us to extend our studies. Some 3.5 years and several hundred patients later, I felt that I had enough knowledge and experience with the drug to submit for publication all of my data which included controlled double-blind and single-blind placebo studies as well as open drug trials. This was accepted by and published in the Journal of the American Medical Association in early 1966. The entire work was divided into two sections; the first dealing with 'clinical pharmacology' and the second dealing with 'clinical therapy'.

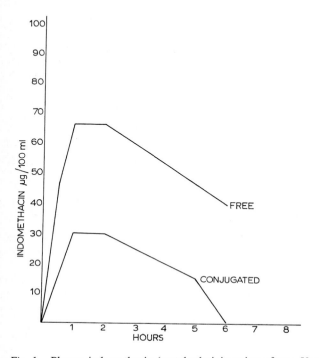

Fig. 1. Plasma indomethacin (rectal administration of two 50 mg capsules).

From these and hundreds of similar reports from all over the world, it was evident that indomethacin had potent anti-rheumatic properties in the human, although dosage limitations were necessary because of distressing side effects. In other words, although a very high rate of benefit could be achieved on doses in the order of 300–400 mg daily, maximum tolerated daily doses could not exceed 200 mg. However, the all important thing was that here at last was a new drug (and a new avenue!) to attack rheumatoid arthritis and the other rheumatic diseases!

A succinct review of the clinical pharmacology of indomethacin should precede our clinical discussions. The drug is now marketed in capsule form containing the highly refined powder which allows for very rapid absorption, plasma levels reaching a peak within an hour and disappearing within 7 hours. It is rapidly conjugated to the glucuronide form as it passes through the liver (Figs. 1 and 2) and in this form it has no apparent clinical activity. The ingested drug may have irritating effects on the gastric mucosa by direct action, presumably dissolving the lipoid protective coating of the gastric lining cells. This would allow reflux of hydrochloric acid through these cells and into the

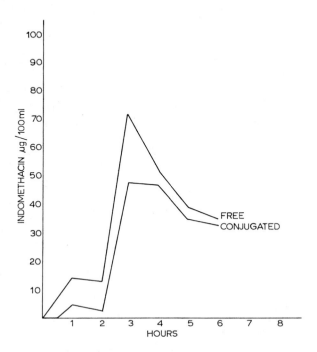

Fig. 2. Plasma indomethacin (rectal administration of two 50 mg capsules).

submucosal layer giving rise to ulcer formation and erosions of blood vessels. In my opinion, there is no good evidence that duodenal ulcers are affected by the drug. Absorption in the upper GI tract is virtually 100%; fecal excretion of free indomethacin is very minimal (Fig. 3). However, large amounts of the

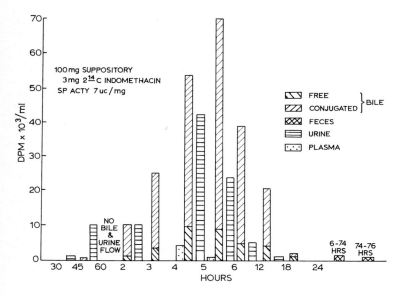

Fig. 3. Pharmacology of indomethacin in man.

glucuronide conjugate are excreted in the stool via the bile. Urinary excretion is large and prompt and mostly in the glucuronide form. In large series of cases, no effect on the bone marrow has been demonstrated, although there have been occasional rare instances reported of idiosyncratic effect. The drug produces strange effects on the sensorium, but these vary greatly with susceptibility. Some individuals have unusually severe headaches, especially in the morning, as well as vertigo, 'muzziness', drowsiness, and sometimes a feeling of being drunk. These effects on sensorium usually disappear quickly with discontinuance of the drug and leave no residual. During the height of these effects, the EEG shows no significant change, the spinal fluid manometrics and content are unaltered, and there are no residual neurologic deficits.

In a rare case the drug apparently produces some diarrhea and bowel irritation. This has been presumed by us to occur in the exceptional individual where indomethacin is excreted by the liver in the free or not fully conjugated form. It must be further presumed that in such exceptional individuals, lower-bowel bleeding would be a possible complication, although accurate documentation is not available. A rare instance of hepatitis has been claimed but in extensive studies by us and others no change in liver enzymes could be documented. There is likewise no ill effect on the kidney.

In summary, indomethacin has a very short half-life in the body and is not cumulative. Its therapeutic and side effects are dissipated within a matter of hours and there are no discernible residuals. From our experience, we concluded that indomethacin is a potent anti-inflammatory, anti-rheumatic agent.

Indomethacin in the long-term therapy of rheumatoid arthritis

S. Teodori and M. Crispo

Istituto di Reumatologia, Rome University, Rome, Italy

The choice of a non-steroidal anti-inflammatory drug to be adopted in the mixed treatment of a chronic disease such as rheumatoid arthritis (RA) must be based not only on the effectiveness of the drug but also on its tolerance. Due to their discontinuous action, anti-inflammatory drugs require almost incessant administration in order to contain within acceptable limits the episodes related to the evolution of the disease. Evidently, a judgement on the properties of such a drug can only be based on experience derived from sufficiently prolonged treatment.

This is the case with indomethacin, the clinical applications of which began in 1962 (Katz et al., 1963; Norcross, 1963; Rothermich, 1963) and which is being widely used by the authors since 1964 in the therapy of rheumatoid arthritics. (See our reports on long-term therapy with indomethacin by Gigante and Teodori (1966) and Capone and Zorzin (1971); the latter report being based on cases studied at the out-patient clinic of our Institute.)

In the present paper we shall report on our experience on a group of cases selected from the extensive material which came to our observation. The group consists exclusively of patients who were repeatedly hospitalized and who, therefore, presented rather severe forms of the disease. In these patients, a steroidal anti-inflammatory drug nearly always had to be added to the basic therapy. The group consisted of 98 subjects, 40 males and 58 females aged from 10 to 75 years, presenting either the classical or the clearly defined form of the disease. There were 12 with involvement of one joint and 86 with involvement of several joints, at different anatomic stages (43 in the Ist and IInd stages and 55 in the IIIrd and IVth stages, according to Steinbrocker). The therapeutic effects were studied from the clinical and bio-humoral standpoints after treatment during periods varying from a minimum of 2 to a maximum of 6 years. The daily dosage of indomethacin was generally between 50 and 150 mg in capsules and/or suppositories. In 86 of the 98 cases, indomethacin was added to a cortisone preparation; the optimal therapeutic program, which we aimed to apply as soon as possible, consisted of a small dose of a steroidal anti-inflammatory drug in the morning (4–8 mg of prednisone or an equivalent dose of another corticosteroid) followed by one 25-mg indomethacin capsule at both main meals; in replacement of or in addition to the evening capsule the treatment included the possibility of administering one 50-mg or one 100-mg suppository before night rest.

Classical criteria of evaluation were adopted, based mainly on objective parameters (importance of joint inflammation, walking time, grip strength) as well as on morning stiffness. We then classified our results as good $(+++)$ fair $(++)$ and middling $(+)$. Bio-humoral tests were performed during the treatment to assess the activity of the disease (sedimentation rate, protein C, electrophoretic analysis of serum proteins) as well as drug tolerance (bilirubinemia, SGOT, SGPT, BSF, urine, azotemia, creatinine clearance, blood cell count, occult intestinal bleeding).

Results

In the 86 patients subjected to mixed treatment, a positive result was recorded in 72% of the cases after 2 years' therapy, in 66% after 3 years, in 60% after 4 years, in 40% after 5 and in 33% after 6 years. An equally positive response was observed in 50% of the subjects treated exclusively with indomethacin for a 2-year period (Fig. 1). Favorable results generally prevail in the forms belonging to the Ist and IInd anatomic stages (Steinbrocker) and having a predominantly inflammatory and exudative nature. The anatomic stage also conditioned the extent of function improvement which is at times not proportional to the improvement of the symptoms of joint inflammation.

Side effects considered globally were noticed in about one-third of the patients studied (Table 1). Side effects involving the nervous system (headache, vertigo, dizziness) are generally transient, they mostly subside spontaneously or following adequate symptomatic therapy, not necessarily with reduction of dosage; exceptionally do they require discontinuance of treatment. The above

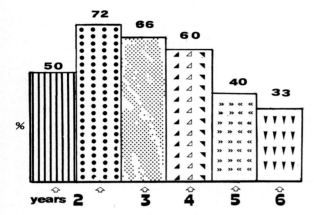

Fig. 1. Percentage of favorable results in 98 cases with regard to type and duration of treatment. Striped column = indomethacin.

TABLE 1

Indomethacin in the long-term therapy of rheumatoid arthritis

Side effects	%	Administration
Gastrointestinal disorders	27.5	Oral
Headache	20.4	Oral or Rectal
Anal itching	8.1	Rectal
Skin rashes	2	Oral or rectal

side effects appear regardless of mode of administration (oral or rectal). Disorders of the gastrointestinal tract (gastralgia, dyspepsia, diarrhea) are more persistent and more frequently require symptomatic treatment or reduction of dosage and, sometimes, discontinuance of treatment. In 2 cases, melaena was observed due to clinically silent gastric or duodenal ulcers and in 4 cases blood was found in the feces. These disorders, naturally, appeared more frequently following oral administration. In 8% of the subjects treated with suppositories, anal-rectal disorders appeared in the form of itching and compulsion. The biohumoral tests indicating activity of the disease showed a trend parallel to the clinical development of the latter in two-thirds of the cases, whereas no significant variations were noted in the tests related to systemic tolerance.

Closing remarks

In drawing final conclusions on prolonged therapy with indomethacin, two general considerations must be taken into account. First, the evaluation of the effectiveness of this drug must allow for the peculiar clinical and evolutionary features of the disease which vary not only according to the different individuals, but also within the same subject. Secondly, the importance of the fundamental contribution which non-steroidal anti-inflammatory drugs can and must bring to the therapy of RA. Evidently, only the cases with the weakest development potential, in other words, a minority of rheumatoid arthritics among those who are hospitalized, can be treated effectively by a therapy based exclusively on such drugs, unless high doses are administered, which is incompatible with long-term treatment. It should not be surprising, therefore, that, in almost all the cases we studied, indomethacin was applied in a mixed treatment with steroidal drugs; however, even in such a therapy, the usefulness of indomethacin is evident because it permits exploitation of the therapeutic synergism of both drugs and, at the same time, reduction of side effects in direct proportion to the dosage applied (Ballabio et al., 1963). To exemplify this, we illustrate, in Figure 2, the case of a 50-year-old man who had been treated by cortisone for 9 years with subsequent development of Cushing's syndrome. The adoption of indomethacin permitted a gradual reduction of the steroid doses with consequent disappearance of the syndrome as well as satisfactory evolution of the disease.

In our case group, the average positive response to mixed therapy was 55%, an undoubtedly appreciable value considering the long duration of the follow-up period, the selection of the cases on the basis of the seriousness of the disease and, above all, the restricting criteria deliberately applied to the evaluation which caused us to consider as positive only the best results obtained ($+++$ and $++$) in order to reduce to a minimum the interference of occasional oscillations in the development of the disease.

The incidence of positive results decreased with time, dropping from 72% after 2 years' treatment to 33% after 6 years. We believe that this should be attributed mainly to the progressive nature of the morbid process rather than to drug resistance caused by habituation. In this connection it is noted that some very rare cases appear from the very beginning to be less sensitive to indomethacin; it is not advisable in these cases to continue beyond a reasonable testing period. In some of these cases, a further attempt at a later date may give favorable results, thus proving the resistance to have been a transient phenomenon connected to the evolution of the disease.

Among the side effects, those affecting the nervous system, particularly

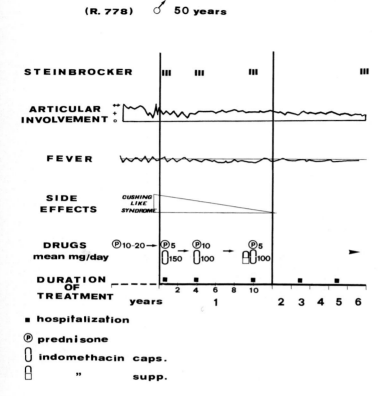

Fig. 2. Reduction of cortisone doses obtained by mixed treatment with indomethacin.

headache, are of little importance; in a long-term, low-dosage treatment such as we have adopted they nearly always have a transient character. More important are the side effects indicating gastrointestinal disorders, as they tend to increase with time. It should be noted that they are common to all anti-inflammatory drugs used orally and over long periods of time and that, in the particular case of mixed treatment, one cannot completely ignore the possible co-responsibility of these steroidal preparations to gastric damage. Such side effects, however, are contained within limits which can be considered as acceptable, especially if they are compared to the therapeutic problem we are called upon to solve. Moreover, except for contraindication of the oral pathway for subjects with gastroduodenal lesions, in most cases the association of an appropriate symptomatic and gastro-protective therapy permitted continuance of treatment with no further inconveniences. In gastric patients, including those suffering from

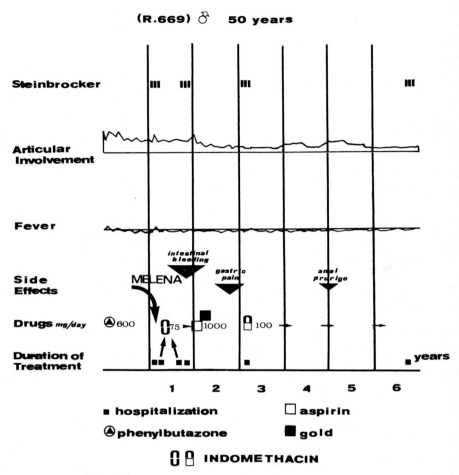

Fig. 3. Tolerance and effectiveness of rectal administration of indomethacin in a patient suffering from duodenal ulcer.

ulcers, the use of suppositories is possible but must be applied with the necessary caution.

Figure 3 describes the case of a 50-year-old man who developed melaena during treatment with phenylbutazone. A duodenal ulcer was diagnosed and the man was subjected to gastroenteroanastomosis. Cautious oral treatment with 75-mg doses of indomethacin resulted in the appearance of blood in the feces. A subsequent tentative treatment with acetylsalicylic acid was discontinued because of gastralgic symptomatology. We then began therapy with indomethacin administered rectally at a daily dose of 100 mg. This proved successful in the control of the disease and was perfectly tolerated by the gastro-intestinal tract for some 4 years except for occasional anal itching. Good tolerance of the rectal pathway was also noted in other cases, such as the 15-year-old girl with juvenile RA who had developed gastric intolerance following mixed treatment with indomethacin, hydroxychloroquine and steroidal drugs (Fig. 4).

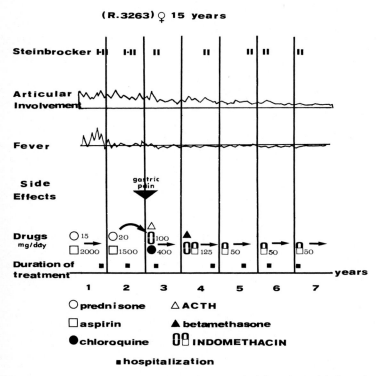

Fig. 4. Tolerance and effectiveness of rectal administration of indomethacin in a case of juvenile rheumatoid arthritis with gastric intolerance.

The absence of clinical phenomena or of laboratory findings expressing liver and kidney parenchymal distress or disorders in the blood system confirms the excellent systemic tolerance of the drug in long-term treatment. In our opinion this feature, together with effectiveness, represents the fundamental property which guarantees indomethacin a prominent position among the non-steroidal anti-inflammatory drugs in the long-term therapy of RA.

References

BALLABIO, C. B., GIRARDI, G., CARUSO, I., CIRLA, E. and COLOMBO, B. (1956): Effetti clinici e metabolici dell'Indomethacin nelle malattie reumatiche. *Reumatismo*, 6, 487.

CAPONE, M. and ZORZIN, L. (1971): Terapia a lungo termine dell'artrite reumatoide con Indomethacin: contributo clinico-statistico. In: *Atti Simposio Inter. Infiamm. e Terapia*, p. 283. Ed. Universo, Firenze.

GIGANTE, D. and TEODORI, S. (1966): Sulla terapia di lunga durata con Indomethacin in reumatologia. *Clin. ter.*, 37, 95.

KATZ, A. M., PEARSON, C. M. and KENNEDY, J. (1963): The anti-rheumatic effects of Indomethacin in rheumatoid arthritis and other rheumatic diseases. *Arthr. and Rheum.*, 6, 281.

NORCROSS, B. M. (1963): Treatment of connective diseases with a new non-steroidal compound (Indomethacin). *Arthr. and Rheum.*, 6, 290.

ROTHERMICH, N. O. (1963): Indomethacin: a new pharmacologic approach to the management of rheumatoid disease. *Arthr. and Rheum.*, 6, 295.

Long-term treatment of rheumatoid arthritis with indomethacin

H. Bröll, G. Tausch and R. Eberl

Department of Rheumatology, City Hospital, Vienna, Austria

As indomethacin differed chemically from the agents then commonly used for the treatment of rheumatic diseases, and knowing the desired and undesired effects of this preparation, we decided – starting in 1965 – on a broad-based treatment of patients from the II Medical Department with Out-Patient Department for Rheumatology of the Vienna Lainz City Hospital with this substance. It proved so tolerable that long-term treatment seemed possible. It also appeared to us that it could be prescribed by the family doctor without any particular permanent control measures being necessary. This was particularly facilitated by the mode of running our out-patient department, as patients suffering from chronic inflammatory diseases of the joints are continually subjected to control checks at 4–6-week intervals after leaving hospital owing to the close cooperation between the family doctor and our department. Only patients who tolerated indomethacin well from the beginning of treatment have been included in this study, all other cases having been excluded (Tables 1, 2 and 3).

1132 patients suffering from definite or classic rheumatoid arthritis, as defined by ARA criteria, were treated with indomethacin. Present findings are based on 1024 patients; 108 patients dropped out in the first 2–4 weeks due to side effects of gastro-intestinal or central nervous origin. Patients with severe cardiac decompensation, liver and renal damage or psychiatric disorders were a priori excluded from this long-term therapy with indomethacin.

TABLE 1

Duration of observation

Years	1	2	3	4	5	6	7	8	9	10	Total
	142	126	24	101	81	76	71	52	30	12	815
	34	25	29	23	27	32	16	12	8	3	209
Total	176	151	153	124	108	108	87	64	38	15	1024

TABLE 2

Patient's age

Age to:	30	40	50	60	70	80	Total
Female	47	65	228	268	195	12	815
Male	16	28	42	84	37	2	209
Total	63	93	270	352	232	14	1024

TABLE 3

Patients' initial grading on the Steinbrocker scale

	Grade				Total
	I	II	III	IV	
	116	455	162	82	815
	31	112	52	14	209
Total	147	567	214	96	1024

Dosage and administration

The level of dosage varied considerably in different patients. Minimum dosage was 25 mg and maximum dosage 200 mg. By 1972, a mean daily dosage of 75 mg had been aimed at, and starting from then an average daily dosage of 150 mg was the aim. If joint exacerbations occurred this average daily dosage was promptly increased to 200 mg. Dyspeptic disorders have been alleviated by rectal administration of the preparation, the patients simultaneously having been given antacids.

As already stated above, only those patients who tolerated indomethacin well have been included in the present long-term study, all other cases having been excluded. 108 patients had to be excluded; 27% of the patients complained about headaches at the beginning of treatment which disappeared on reduction of dosage without additional therapy.

The following laboratory investigations were made first at intervals of 2–4 weeks, then 6–8 weeks and, in patients on therapy for more than 1 year, at 3-monthly intervals: erythrocyte sedimentation rate, blood and urine status, serum C-reactive protein and serum lability test, transaminase determination, renal function tests, Latex fixation (Singer-Plotz), haemagglutination by the Waaler-Rose method. Detailed ophthalmological examinations were performed on all patients treated with indomethacin for more than 5 years by the staff of the Eye Department of Vienna Lainz City Hospital, because of the report by Burns (1968) of ophthalmologic disturbances.

Assessment of the clinical state of rheumatoid arthritis was based both on ARA criteria and those developed by Fähndrich (1952) and Halhuber et al. (1955).

Results

Based on the evaluation criteria we considered it a very good result if indomethacin alone was sufficient for a therapeutic effect. It was considered a good result if in the observation period additional anti-rheumatic medication became necessary in flare-up situations. Permanently necessary additional therapy was regarded as a poor result. Patients in the last-named group throughout belonged to stages II and IV according to Steinbrocker.

A very good therapeutic effect was demonstrated in 298 (26.3%) patients. A good response was confirmed in 684 (60.4%) patients, and an adequate effect in 42 (3.7%) patients. No toxic influence on either the liver or the kidneys was shown in the course of this long-term study. In addition, no changes in the blood picture were observed during treatment.

Ophthalmologic examination revealed no cases of corneal deposition, and neither visual nor fundal changes. One patient who had been treated for 2½ years with 75 mg indomethacin had a right-sided haemorrhage involving the retina and vitreous humour which we did not associate with the medication.

One patient, who had been treated for 2 years with indomethacin, developed a florid duodenal ulcer. Anamnestically such an ulcer had first been confirmed 6 years before. Oral therapy (150 mg/day) was changed to rectal administration, and 2 months later the ulcer healed up again under ulcer therapy. Two other patients developed florid ulcers after 12 months. They were treated with 5 mg prednisolone and 150 mg indomethacin daily. The oral administration was also changed to rectal application.

Starting in 1971, clinical tolerance was studied in 651 patients who were subjected to a basic treatment with chloroquine, gold or D-penicillamine. 425 patients received chloroquine, 163 aqueous gold salts, and 63 D-penicillamine. No interference phenomena between the individual preparations could be observed. The clinical tolerance was the same as with the above long-term study.

References

BURNS, C. A. (1968): *Amer. J. Ophthal.*, *66*, 825.
FÄHNDRICH, W. H. (1952): *J. rheumat. Res.*, *11*, 36.
HALHUBER, M., HAUS, E. and INAMA, K. (1955): *J. rheumat. Res.*, *14*, 159.

Indomethacin in the treatment of the lumbar disc syndrome

A. Ciocci

Istituto di Reumatologia, University of Rome, Italy

The lumbar disc or lumbar sacral syndrome includes the clinical patterns which (Gigante et al., 1972) manifest as acute lumbago, chronic lumbago or sciatica, the aetiopathogenesis of which is a primary disorder of the intervertebral disc. The common pathogenic cause of these different patterns is proved by the not infrequent occurrence of lumbago and sciatica at different times in the same patient.

Anatomically, both acute and chronic lumbago are caused by the infiltration of the nucleus pulposus into the altered structures of the annulus which, as is well known, is innervated by the fibres of Luschka's nerve. Sciatica is caused by disc-posterior root pressure; caused by herniation of the disc. We need not mention that the disc-posterior root pressure can also cause simple clinical patterns of acute or chronic lumbago.

Although it can be said that, anatomically, primary disc distress is the cause of clinical patterns of chronic and acute lumbago, it must be emphasized that often no clinical pattern (i.e. no painful episodes) occurs in the presence of disc alterations clearly evident by X-ray. This means that disc alteration alone may sometimes not be sufficient to bring about a clinical pattern; for the latter to appear, an inflammatory episode – oedematous or congestive – is necessary, causing damage to the structures involved in the disc alteration.

In view of this inflammatory component, which is the same as that found in clinically evident osteoarthritis, we thought it interesting to study the use of indomethacin in the lumbar disc syndrome from a somewhat different angle than the one adopted by other authors in their research on similar case groups. This drug which, as is well known, also possesses a secondary, but important, analgesic property, became particularly useful as an anti-rheumatic drug thanks to its primary powerful anti-inflammatory action.

The group we examined consisted of 225 patients of different ages and of both sexes. Of the cases with involvement of the disc apparent on X-ray, 58 had acute lumbago, 50 chronic lumbago, and 56 sciatica. The other 61 had chronic lumbago without involvement of the disc but with osteophytosis.

We adopted different criteria such as X-rays, anamnestic data (duration of disease), anagraphical data, clinical data (type and duration of clinical pattern), etc. to differentiate patients with chronic lumbago with disc damage from patients with chronic lumbago due to spondylarthritis, a differentiation which was perhaps more convenient than realistic.

We administered to all patients doses of indomethacin varying from 75 to 200 mg per day for 14–28 days. After at least 7 days treatment, when the clinical pattern required it, other analgesic drugs or corticosteroids were associated. Several patients were subjected at the same time to physico-kinetic and massage therapy. All patients were made to rest on hard beds. Subjects with gastro-duodenal symptoms were excluded from this treatment.

It should be pointed out that many factors can influence the evaluation of results: the different ages of patients, the duration of disease, the impossibility of a strict classification of the various disorders; for example, we do not know whether we should have classified as acute lumbago patients who suffered other episodes of lumbago in the recent past. Apart from this example, there might be other causes for doubt as to the precision of our classification of cases into four groups, namely acute lumbago, chronic lumbago, sciatica (all with disc involvement apparent on X-ray) and lumbago from spondylarthritis. In our opinion, however, this classification is sufficient for the purposes of our present contribution.

We classified our results as 'none', 'modest', 'good', 'excellent', on the basis of the efficacy (reduction of painful symptomatology, both subjective and objective and functional improvement). If we consider the results classified (Table 1) as 'good' and 'excellent' as 'positive', we see that a high percentage of these results was obtained in patients with chronic lumbago (90%) and with lumbago from spondylarthritis (78%). The incidence of positive results was considerably lower in patients with acute lumbago or with sciatica, 52% and 50% respectively.

Our results do not differ substantially, in percentages, from those obtained by Rubens-Duval et al. (1967). In a group of 38 sciatica cases they obtained complete or nearly complete recovery in 42% (16 cases) and they either ob-

TABLE 1

Results

Diagnosis	No. of cases	Effect				Positive results (%)
		None	Modest	Good	Excellent	
Acute lumbago	58	12	16	18	12	52
Chronic lumbago	50	—	5	15	30	90
Sciatica	56	9	19	22	6	50
Lumbago from spondylarthritis	61	4	12	18	27	78

tained an improvement (12 cases) or failed (10 cases) in the remainder. However, at a round table held during the First Latin Congress on Rheumatology last November at which I was also present, Villiaumey gave us some data related to a group of cases in which he had differentiated (as we have) patients with an exclusively degenerative pattern from those presenting an acute pattern of lumbar distress. These data were practically identical to ours. Our results are also similar to the ones achieved by our colleagues at Prof. Ballabio's Department of Rheumatology at Milan University (Fantini and Colombo, 1971) if one allows for the difference in approach of both contributions.

How should we interpret the different results achieved in the four groups we have considered? In our opinion, the explanation could lie in the different inflammatory components which cause the appearance and the duration of the various clinical patterns belonging to the lumbar disc syndrome. The importance attributed, particularly by French and Italian authors, to the inflammatory component in the pathogenesis of some patterns of disc distress is thus supported by therapeutic evidence. Robecchi clearly stated in this connection that 'residual inflammatory reactions, however slight, would be the cause of protracted pain in chronic lumbago'. We believe that, in the light of more modern views on 'clinically evident' arthrosis, it is also possible to emphasize the importance of the reactive-inflammatory component in the pathogenesis of the clinical pattern of 'lumbago from spondylarthritis'. It is evident that the episodes of exacerbation of painful symptoms in a subject with spondylarthritis can only be due to a dynamic inflammatory process occurring in addition to the static osteo-degenerative basic pattern. If these pathogenetic assumptions are correct, they can provide a logical explanation for the differences in the results we have obtained.

As far as the low incidence of positive results in cases of acute lumbago is concerned, it must be remembered that the element responsible for acute lumbago is now considered to be a primary structural degeneration of the disc, characterized by the migration of the nucleus into the nearest structures of the annulus. Thus it would seem possible to maintain that the acute lumbago episode is due more to immediate distress due to irritation or compression of the nerve endings in the disc than to damage mediated by oedema following inflammation of the structures involved.

The low incidence of positive results in cases of sciatica has, in our opinion, two causes. First, although we recognize, with De Sèze, the importance of the irritation-inflammation component of disc-posterior root damage, we also believe that in some cases, or in some stages of the development, the clinical pattern is caused or largely caused by primary damage to the posterior root due to mechanical constriction exerted by the herniated disc. Secondly, in patients suffering from sciatica – and this is probably a more important consideration – the painful component is in itself much stronger than in patients belonging to other groups, so that indomethacin, which does not have a predominantly analgesic action, does not give qualitatively excellent results.

During our trial we obviously also studied the possible occurrence of various disorders which could be attributed to the drug administered. Fairly frequently – in 19% of the cases (43) – the patients complained of slight disorders related to the central nervous system (headache, vertigo) or to the digestive system. 28 other patients had to discontinue therapy with indomethacin following serious disorders related mainly to the gastrointestinal tract (Table 2). The incidence of phenomena which required discontinuance of treatment was 10.1% of the total group treated (253 patients). These data do not differ from those reported by other authors, sometimes on the basis of much larger case groups.

We conclude that the results obtained in our study can be considered on the

TABLE 2

Cases which required discontinuance of treatment (total of 253 patients)

Side effects	No. of cases	%
Gastric disorders	14	5.5
Nervous symptoms	8	3.1
Associated symptoms (nervous, gastric, etc.)*	4	1.5
Total	28	10.1

No cases of gastric or duodenal ulcers, enterorrhagia, or cholecyst perforation were seen.
*Headache, vertigo, confusion, drowsiness, epigastralgia, nausea, pyrosis, dyspepsia, oedema, skin rash, itching.

whole as clearly positive and as evidence of the usefulness of indomethacin in this type of disorder. The different incidence of positive results in the various groups of patients indicates, on the one hand, the anti-inflammatory qualities of this drug and, on the other, the specificity and the complexity of its pharmacological properties.

We can assume – given the different behaviour of the drug with regard to the same disease according to the site of the disease itself – that the drug is active on different links of the pathogenetic chain which leads to pain in the motor system. Researchers should therefore direct their attention to this area. Thus, perhaps, a valid explanation could be given for the different therapeutic effects of indomethacin in, for example, osteoarthritis of the hip, in which, as we know, brilliant results are obtained, and gonarthritis, where positive results account for only 40%.

References

FANTINI, F. and COLOMBO, B. (1971): Impiego dell'Indometacina nel trattamento dell'osteoartrosi e di altre affezioni reumatologiche minori. In: *Atti Simposio Internazionale sull'infiammazione e sua terapia, Firenze, 1971*, pp. 303–308.

GIGANTE, D., CASTAGNOLI, M. and TEODORI S. (1972): Clinica dell'artrosi. In: *Atti XVI Giorn. Med. Montecatini*, 1972, pp. 85–177.

RUBENS-DUVAL, A., VILLIAUMEY, J. and DUROUX, P. (1967): Emploi de l'Indométacine dans le traitement de la lombosciatique aigüe. *Rev. Rhum., 34*, 177.

Indomethacin in the treatment of ankylosing spondylitis

D. Focan-Henrard and P. Franchimont

Department of Rheumatology, Medical Institute, University of Liège, Belgium

Indomethacin has been regarded since its introduction into clinical practice as one of the most promising of the new, non-steroidal anti-inflammatory agents, especially for the treatment of patients with ankylosing spondylitis and gout. Now that the product has been in widespread use for 10 years, it seems interesting to draw up a balance and determine whether it has lived up to the hopes rheumatologists had of it. Although in a number of diseases its role is largely that of one supportive therapy among many, in certain rheumatic

TABLE 1

Results obtained by various authors in patients with spondylitis treated with indomethacin

	0	+	++	+++	Total
Delbarre et al. (1965)	3	2	9	16	31
Gigante (1965)	1	2	3	9	15
Dudley Hart and Boardman (1965)	9	1	6	16	32
De Sèze et al. (1965)	6	4	5	8	25
Doury (1967)	3		9	9	21
Calabro and Amante (1968)	0	2	5	21	28
Franchimont and Van Cauwenberge (1968)	9		24		33
Bloch-Michel and Rouaud (1972)	10		9	24	43
Hiemeyer (1972)	1	2		8	11

0 = failure, + = good results, ++ = very good results, +++ = excellent results.

diseases it is remarkably effective, as confirmed by sustained, controlled tests. First among these diseases is ankylosing spondylitis. Calabro (1975) even states that if indomethacin does not cause a significant attenuation of the pain, the diagnosis of spondylitis may well be wrong. Table 1 lists the results obtained by a number of authors who have tried indomethacin in spondylitis; admittedly, comparison is difficult since different authors have applied different criteria of evaluation. It is nevertheless clear that on the whole, very good and excellent results have been obtained in the majority: of the 239 cases listed in this table, 75.7% have exhibited excellent or very good results.

Criteria of evaluation

Subjective criteria

Pain. When we review the various criteria that have been applied to assess the efficacy of the product, it is immediately clear that indomethacin acts first of all on the pain component of the disease; we find, in fact, that the subjective action on the pain is very frequent (it is encountered in 70 to 80% of the cases), pronounced (complete freedom from pain may be achieved) and rapid (in a few days).

Morning stiffness. The action on morning stiffness (the inflammatory component) is also pronounced, and most patients report improved mobility on getting up, with reduced duration of stiffness: from 63 to 41 minutes in the series of De Sèze et al. (1965). More particularly, it appears that a 100 mg suppository or an oral dose of 100 mg given at night results in good mitigation of nocturnal pain and, owing to its fairly sustained effect, attenuation of morning stiffness (Huskisson and Dudley Hart, 1972).

Objective criteria

Functional capacity. When we consider the objective clinical criteria of efficacy, i.e. in the first place the determination of functional capacity, the results are slightly less excellent. Nevertheless, in a considerable proportion of the cases we observe improvement of the functional capacity determined by measuring the finger-floor distance, the occiput-wall distance, the chest expansion, etc. Franchimont and Van Cauwenberge (1968) observed 72% with subjective improvement with indomethacin as against only 50% with objective improvement, in 33 patients followed up for at least 2 years.

Biological criteria. The effect of indomethacin on biological criteria is even less. This effect is rather inconstant: in almost one-half of the cases, the sedimentation rate appears to be little affected by the therapy. Also, there is no parallel to be observed between the clinical evolution and the results of inflammation tests. However, in this connection it should be kept in mind that in 30 to 40% of cases, the inflammation tests are never abnormal (Franchiment and Van Cauwenberge, 1968). In the trial of indomethacin by De Sèze et al. (1965), the sedimentation rate decreased in 10 out of 25 cases.

Factors that influence the effect of indomethacin

When we consider the effects of indomethacin in relation to the stage of the disease, we find that the earlier the stage, the more favourable are the effects; also, the action of the product is better in the acute phases of the disease. In the advanced stages of the disease, indomethacin is less effective.

We may add that individual susceptibility varies greatly. In patients responding favourably, the dosage to which they respond may differ very much from one individual to another. The initial dose often amounts to 100 mg at least, but may be as high as 200 or even 300 mg. Maintenance treatment sometimes requires daily doses as large as 100 mg or more, but often 25 mg per day, or even every other day, will be enough to keep the symptoms under control. In certain cases it even seems permissible to attempt short periods of withdrawal.

In regard to the dose distribution, Huskisson and Dudley Hart (1972) have reported that administration of one dose of 100 mg indomethacin at night results in good attenuation of nocturnal pain and, owing to the sustained effect, reduced stiffness on awakening.

It should be noted in this connection that the effects of indomethacin in principle only last as long as the product is administered: in the vast majority of cases, discontinuation of the drug is rapidly followed by a return of the pain and the inflammatory symptoms.

The effects of indomethacin on the long-term evolution of ankylosing spondylitis

Whereas indomethacin leads to improvement of the subjective symptomatology of pain, it does not appear to affect the long-term evolution of the disease: in the series studied by Franchimont and Van Cauwenberge (1968), the objective tests in 22% of the patients revealed a reduction of spinal mobility or of chest expansion in spite of subjective improvement in patients who were followed up for a period of 2 years.

The radiological aspects were not influenced by the treatment either: patients who were followed up for several years exhibited aggravation of the radiological picture in spite of attenuation of pain.

The effects of indomethacin on the extra-spinal manifestations of spondylitis

The effects of indomethacin on the peripheral, articular manifestations of spondylitis appear to be less than the effects on the spinal symptoms, even though in our personal trials the preparation appeared to alleviate nocturnal pain and morning stiffness in the majority of cases.

As regards the effects on the internal organs, it is almost unanimously agreed in the literature that indomethacin exerts no effect on the cardiovascular lesions. Where iritis is concerned, opinions are more divided, but most authors agree that the effect is slight at best. However, in the few cases that we have observed personally, the impression was gained that treatment with indomethacin alone resulted in a significant decrease of the frequency of this painful ocular complication.

Side effects

The strongest argument against the routine use of indomethacin in the treatment of patients with spondylitis is the high frequency of side effects and of signs of intolerance.

In some series, the incidence of side effects was as high as 50 to 60%. The most frequent manifestations are neurological (headache, dizziness, drowsiness) or digestive (anorexia, epigastric pain, etc.).

Some patients exhibit only transient manifestations in the early stages of the disease (22.6% in the series of De Sèze at al. (1965)), but, in most cases, the side effects persist throughout treatment (52% in the same series).

On the other hand, it is only in a small proportion of the cases (5%) that these side effects necessitate interruption of the treatment; since the patients clearly experience good results, they accept the side effects, which in any case are benign as a rule. Also, between indomethacin and phenylbutazone, another preparation effective against spondylitis, there is not necessarily cross-intolerance, and, since the same holds true where the therapeutic effects are concerned, we have at our disposal two preparations that may easily be interchanged to the patients' greater benefit.

In our experience, the incidence of side effects can be reduced considerably by reducing the doses, altering their distribution, by administration of the drug prior to meals and by associated administration of gastroprotective substances. In particular, with doses smaller than 100 mg we have only very rarely encountered any neurological side effects. The impression has also been gained that side effects may be attenuated by administering the main dose at bedtime.

Conclusions

After some 10 years' use of indomethacin, we believe that it is one of the drugs of choice in the treatment of ankylosing spondylitis.

The excellent efficacy of the drug is comparable to that of phenylbutazone. In many cases, it may be administered without objection for very long periods of time (several years). Moreover, the preparation is free from the dangerous side effects (on the liver, the kidneys, and the blood) that have been attributed to phenylbutazone.

However, in contrast to the very good effects on the pain and the inflamatory symptoms, the drug appears to exert much less effect on the long-term evolution of the disease. Its effect on the basic pathogenesis is only very slight.

Finally, there is a very high degree of individual variability where therapeutic efficacy and tolerance are concerned; however, there is no constant cross-relationship with the efficacy and tolerance of phenylbutazone, so that good effects may be obtained with indomethacin where the pyrazole derivatives have failed, or vice versa.

These few reservations do not detract from the fact that in many cases of ankylosing spondylitis, indomethacin alleviates rheumatic attacks and reduces their incidence, sometimes to nil over very long periods of time, so that it facilitates rehabilitation and treatment aimed at prevention of spinal deformities, and allows the patients to lead a normal social and occupational life, a result that is the more important in that the disease predominantly strikes young, active persons.

References

BLOCH-MICHEL, H. and ROUAUD, J. P. (1972): Traitement des pelvispondylites par l'indomethacine. Résultats cliniques de traitements au long cours. In: *Symposium International sur l'Inflammation et son Traitement, Florence, 1971*, p. 185. S.P.E.I., Paris.
CALABRO, J. J. (1975): Long-term reappraisal of indomethacin. *Drug Ther.*, 5 (2), 46.
CALABRO, J. J. and AMANTE, C. M. (1968): Indomethacin in ankylosing spondylitis. *Arthr. and Rheum.*, 11/1, 56.

DELBARRE, F., AMOR, B. and BROUILLET, H. (1965): Un nouvel anti-inflammatoire: l'indomethacine. *Sem. Hôp.*, *8*, 429.

DE SÈZE, S., RYCKEWAERT, A., KAHN, M. F. and SOLNICA, J. (1965): Résultats d'un essai contrôlé de l'indomethacine en rheumatologie. *Rev. Rhum.*, *32/12*, 769.

DOURY, P. (1967): La place de l'indomethacine dans le traitement de 6 spondylarthrite ankylosante: à propos de 21 observations. *Thérapeutique*, *44/10*, 631.

DUDLEY HART, F. and BOARDMAN, P. L. (1965): Indomethacin and phenylbutazone: a comparison. *Brit. Med. J.*, *8*, 1281.

FRANCHIMONT, P. and VAN CAUWENBERGE, H. (1968): Notre expérience de certains médicaments utilisés dans la spondylarthrite ankylosante. *J. belge Rhum. Méd. phys.*, *23*, 5.

GIGANTE, D. (1965): L'indomethacin mella térapia della gotta e della spondilite anchilosante. In: *Terapia Antireumatica nonsteroida, Turin, June, 1965*. Minerva Medica.

HIEMEYER, V. (1972): Action antiinflammatoire et analgésique de l'indomethacin dans les arthropathies inflammatoires, le cancer, la maladie de Hodgkin et la leucémie myéloide chronique. In: *Symposium International sur l'Inflammation et son Traitement, Florence, 1971*, p. 171. S.P.E.I., Paris.

HUSKISSON, E. C. and DUDLEY HART, F. (1972): The use of indomethacin and aloxiprin at night. *Practitioner*, *208*, 248.

IIIB. *Past, present and future of indomethacin*

Chairman   S. de Sèze
Co-chairman E. C. Huskisson

Introduction

S. de Sèze

Service de Rhumatologie, Centre Viggo Petersen, Hôpital Lariboisière, Paris, France

With regard to the Session I have the honour of presenting – Past, Present and Future of Indomethacin – I think that three fundamental dates can help us to answer the three questions: what is important in the past?; what is the present status?; and what are the perspectives for the future? The three dates I refer to are 1965, 1971 and 1975.

In 1965, after three years of continuous experimental work, indomethacin was presented, and I would like to remember the paper by Charley Smith and that by Diver, who showed the therapeutic value of indomethacin (compared to steroids) in rheumatoid arthritis. This new agent soon appeared very useful in the treatment of inflammatory diseases of the joints, even though less effective than steroids.

Of the first works published on the therapeutic properties of indomethacin, I would recall the study by Recordier and those by Michote and Dixon (confirmed by Recordier), who showed that this anti-inflammatory agent was particularly active against pain in degenerative joint disease of the hip (in 60 cases out of 68).

At that time, this pharmacological activity in the course of osteoarthritis of the hip was widely discussed. It seemed at the very least odd that an anti-inflammatory agent should be the best treatment for pain in degenerative joint disease. However, this pain relief appeared so marked that some authors raised the possibility that this alleviation encouraged patients affected by degenerative joint disease of the hips and treated with indomethacin to perform extensive physical activity, thus worsening the anatomic status of the hip joints. We do not agree with this paradoxical opinion.

In 1965, Isemein reported that indomethacin was very efficient in the treatment of gout; the same observation was soon confirmed by others, particularly Hawthorn.

I would like to close this review of 1965 by discussing two papers published by two of the most distinguished clinics in Paris. The first of these studies was by Professor Coste, who concluded that indomethacin was an excellent antirheumatic agent and that in the future it would be one of the main anti-inflammatory agents used in the treatment of rheumatic diseases. It was not easy to predict this success in 1965, and it was a brilliant prediction.

The other study was performed by Professor M. Khan (Rheumatologic Clinic of Lariboisiere) and myself; we concluded that indomethacin was a pharmacologic agent with a wide range of application in the field of rheumatology. Thus, in 1965 the first clinical experiences were reported with great hopes.

During the following five years, from 1965 to 1971, rheumatologists from all over the world used this anti-inflammatory agent, which reawakened interest in rheumatic inflammation and its treatment, fifteen years after the advent of cortisone and ten years after the synthesis of phenylbutazone. Interest in this subject became very great and widespread all over the world, so that a large number of papers on indomethacin were published; the culmination of this outstanding work was the International Symposium held in Florence in 1971. Most of you, I am sure, will remember that experience.

During the Symposium held in Florence in 1971 – and this is the second date I mentioned when starting my talk – most of the research workers engaged in this field raised the possibility of objective parameters of inflammation, to evaluate the effect of indomethacin on a more scientific basis. Dryle, Hiemeyer, Anselm, Fricke and Pawlowski proposed a series of procedures, more or less complicated, to be applied to future studies on indomethacin; in this way, results of these studies would be more objective and clearer.

On the other hand, studies were performed to understand the true mechanism of the pharmacological activity of indomethacin; after some years of clinical experience, it was no longer sufficient to know only that indomethacin was active. The studies reported by Wagner on the mechanism of action of anti-inflammatory non-steroidal agents, and the paper by Brouillet made a significant contribution to this problem and brought the problem of the anti-inflammatory properties of indomethacin to an experimental level.

Of course, these studies of physiology and pharmacodynamics gave a solid base to the clinical works presented at the Florence Symposium – even though six years afterwards – concerning the results obtained by rheumatologists from twenty countries with indomethacin in the treatment of inflammatory rheumatic disease, gout, degenerative joint disease, particularly of the hip, periarthritis of the shoulder, sciatica, and sports trauma. In 1975, ten years after the synthesis of indomethacin, we are just celebrating this occurrence. Ten years is quite a long time for any agent which has little or no inherent pharmacological powers; such agents go out of common clinical use despite publicity. In contrast, the interest for indomethacin has been constantly growing and it has now become an agent currently prescribed by many physicians, not only by rheumatologists.

I am sure that the place of indomethacin in the treatment of rheumatic diseases will be more clearly defined by this Symposium on Inflammatory Arthropathies. Moreover, it will indicate the future role of the industry which produces indomethacin.

This Symposium has given us the opportunity of evaluating the clinical trials with indomethacin which have been conducted during the last ten years, and I would recall the presentation by Rothermich on long-term tolerance, the studies by Rothermich and Haslock on the treatment of rheumatoid arthritis, by Le Quesne on degenerative joint disease of the hip, by Ciocci on discal degeneration, by Dudley Hart and Franchimont on ankylosing spondylitis, by Bacon on gout, and by A. Peltier on the painful shoulder syndrome.

But in the Programme we also find general subjects such as the cytology of inflammation, microcrystalline inflammation, the role of complement in inflammation, and the unitary theory of inflammation. In other words, basic studies on inflammation which have nothing to do with indomethacin.

It is a pleasure to see from this programme that the large laboratories of the pharmacological industry, particularly Merck, Sharp and Dohme, have understood that it is in their interest not only to sell as much as possible of the drugs they develop, but also to support – inside and outside the industry – research which may one day bring substantial progress in rheumatology, and to help post-degree training, which is so important for the diffusion in the scientific world of the new data acquired on rheumatology. Merck, Sharp and Dohme laboratories accepted these priorities, so that I am sure I echo the opinions of most rheumatologists when I say that they really serve rheumatology well.

Indomethacin in rheumatoid arthritis. A review

Ian Haslock

Department of Rheumatology, South Tees Health District, Middlesborough, United Kingdom

The treatment of rheumatoid arthritis is not simply a matter of giving drugs. Our role as rheumatologists is becoming increasingly complicated as we have to co-ordinate the efforts of many other workers in providing optimum treatment for our patients. Despite the need for increasing knowledge of many other fields our own direct therapeutic role is largely concerned with drugs. As no cure for rheumatoid arthritis exists we have to evaluate the benefits and dangers of each drug individually and must always remember we are dealing with a disease which may last a lifetime. Because of this we tend to be rather conservative in our prescribing and this conservatism is justified by the presence in our clinics of patients treated with corticosteroids in their heyday, patients who now suffer more from the adverse effects of therapy than from their rheumatoid disease.

Despite these reminders of the consequences of miscalculation, simple conservatism is not a sufficient reason for adhering to traditional prescribing patterns if more appropriate remedies are now available. It is within this context that I wish to review the use of indomethacin, which has become one of the most widely prescribed drugs used in the treatment of rheumatoid arthritis. I have used three broad headings for this review. Firstly, is the drug effective in the short term? Secondly, is its effectiveness maintained for the long periods necessary in treating rheumatoid arthritis and thirdly is it safe and well tolerated during these long periods?

Early trials of indomethacin were designed to demonstrate its superiority to placebo and to compare its efficacy with that of high dosage aspirin therapy and with phenylbutazone. I shall consider these first, and then consider comparisons with the newer preparations which are appearing on the market with increasing frequency. Hart and Boardman (1963) employed cross-over techniques to show that substitution of placebo for indomethacin caused a rapid rebound of symptoms in rheumatoid patients. They were also able to demonstrate a reduction in p.i.p. joint swelling during indomethacin treatment, this being considered good evidence of anti-inflammatory effect. Not all placebo trials have produced similar results. The A.R.A. compared 71 patients on indomethacin with 65 on placebo (Co-operating Clinics Committee, 1967). Their finding of no difference between the two therapies obtained wide publicity. The reason is simple. Each of the participating clinics continued to use aspirin in their usual fashion during the course of the trial. In fact, aspirin consumption decreased in the patients taking indomethacin but not in the controls. Decrease in aspirin consumption was shown by McGuire and Wright (1971) to be a valuable index of efficacy in a clinical trial and it is widely used as such, especially in the Lansbury index (Lansbury, 1956). We now also know that co-administration of aspirin and indomethacin introduces the problem of a pharmacokinetic interaction which significantly lowers plasma indomethacin levels (Jeremy and Towson, 1970; Rubin et al., 1973).

Turning to comparison of indomethacin and aspirin, the in-patient study by Pitkeathly and his colleagues was carefully analysed to eliminate the effects of hospitalisation on the patients' disease. They found that p.i.p. joint size was reduced to a similar degree by both therapies and that grip strength improved rather more on indomethacin. Their overall conclusion was that the anti-inflammatory effect of 100 mg indomethacin and 4 g aspirin were comparable (Pitkeathly et al., 1966). Our own comparison of indomethacin and aspirin took the form of an in-patient double-blind cross-over trial of 100 mg indomethacin against 5 g micro-encapsulated aspirin (Haslock et al., 1975). We found that, irrespective of treatment order reduction of pain was more rapid during the first week of the trial than the second, reflecting the effect of hospital treatment. Summation of the two treatment periods showed pain relief to be similar with the two preparations and grip strength was also affected similarly by the two drugs. Morning stiffness was of considerable interest to us as it was thought that the 2-g dose of sustained release aspirin which we gave at night might be more effective by morning than the 50-mg night dose of indomethacin. In fact there was no difference between the two treatment regimes. We did find that the patient's ESR rose on indomethacin despite clinical improvement. This phenomenon has been observed many times but it still disturbs rheumatologists who have been brought up to think of the ESR as the one reliable objective test of efficacy available to them. The search for alternative objective tests is exercising workers in many parts of the world, one of the most active groups in this respect being that at the Centre for Rheumatic Disease at Glasgow. It is of some interest to complete our study of indomethacin and salicylates by examining the results of comparisons of these two drugs with each other and with placebo using the battery of tests devised by that unit (Dick et al., 1970). As is seen from Table 1, these show the articular index significantly improved by

TABLE 1

Comparison of indomethacin, sodium salicylate and placebo

	Corrected mean scores		
	Indomethacin	Salicylate	Placebo
Articular index	21.6	25.5	41.1
Knee score	5.3	6.0	9.2
Joint size	48.6	48.0	51.6
Grip strength	68.2	60.1	48.2
Xenon T$\frac{1}{2}$	38.2	33.0	20.9
Tc peak counts	15,400	21,200	28,700

(After Dick et al., 1970.)

both drugs, 100 mg indomethacin being marginally better than 5 g sodium salicylate. Their knee scores showed similar results. Joint size was not significantly reduced by either treatment but grip strength showed improvement by both active therapies. Xenon clearance from the knee joint was only marginally improved by the active drugs, but Technecium peak counts over the knee showed a highly significant difference between active and placebo therapy and in this test the superiority of indomethacin over aspirin approached statistical significance (p $\doteq$ 0.1). The authors concluded that the findings in their study were in agreement with the suggestion that the anti-inflammatory action of indomethacin is greater than that of aspirin.

I have spent quite a long time comparing indomethacin with salicylates because aspirin is still described as 'the yardstick against which all other agents should be measured'. The results of that measurement shows 100 mg indomethacin to be at least as effective as high dose salicylate therapy.

Comparisons with other analgesic/anti-inflammatory agents must be more brief. I shall summarise the studies against phenylbutazone by highlighting one trial which gives results that are typical but which was carried out with an unusual degree of care because it was designed as a vehicle for assessment of clinical trial methodology as well as of the drugs concerned. After a 2-week period during which the patients' disease activity had to be stable, Wright and co-workers (1969) compared the effects of indomethacin, phenylbutazone and placebo in 24 out-patients with rheumatoid arthritis. The trial was a double-blind, double placebo cross-over and the dose of medication was increased during the appropriate periods from 100 to 300 mg phenylbutazone and from 50 to 150 mg indomethacin. Supplementary aspirin was used as required and the amount taken used as a measurement within the trial.

Indomethacin was shown to be significantly superior to placebo in reduction of pain and aspirin consumption but, of more importance in our present context, it was also shown to be statistically indistinguishable from phenylbutazone in terms of activity measured by pain, restriction of movement, morning stiffness, time to onset of fatigue, grip strength and aspirin need. It is also interesting that both side effects and drop-outs were minimised by the use of an incremental dose schedule. This was also true of the study we carried out of indomethacin against the turpenepyrazole compound feprazone (Haslock et al., 1976). We used an introductory period on paracetamol, and minimised interactions between anti-inflammatory agents by forbidding aspirin during the trial. 300 mg of feprazone daily was compared with 75 rising to 150 mg indomethacin in a double-blind cross-over trial. Joint size did not alter during the study period, but both therapies produced a significant improvement in pain (p < 0.005), morning stiffness (p < 0.005) and grip strength (p < 0.001) when compared with the paracetamol run-in period. The patients showed significant overall improvement during the course of the trial with no difference between the two drug regimes. No drop-outs occurred because of side effects during the indomethacin periods in this trial, but this was not so when we attempted to compare an initial dose of 150 mg indomethacin daily with 500 mg naproxen in out-patients with rheumatoid arthritis (Haslock et al., 1973). Results from the first 11 patients in this study only are available, but 3 of these dropped out early in the course of indomethacin treatment because of the occurrence of side effects. A similar study of 150 mg indomethacin against 500 mg naproxen has been completed in Norway (Kogstad, 1973). Twenty-six patients with rheumatoid arthritis completed this double-blind cross-over trial, and the two therapies were found to be statistically similar in terms of joint scores, morning stiffness, time to fatigue, walking time and grip strength. Two other trials totalling 65 patients have shown similar results, 500 mg naproxen being comparable with 150 mg indomethacin in short-term studies (D'Omézon, 1973; Szanto, 1974). More recently two doses of naproxen, 750 mg and 500 mg daily, have been compared with indomethacin 100 mg and placebo in a cross-over fashion (Hernandez et al., 1975). Both drugs proved significantly superior to placebo but no significant differences were observed between them.

Naproxen is one of the series of propionic acid derivatives which are the most recently introduced group of analgesic/anti-inflammatory agents. The earliest of these was ibuprofen but as this is at best a moderate analgesic and mild anti-inflammatory agent it does not contribute significantly to the management of rheumatoid arthritis. Two newer members of this class are fenoprofen and ketoprofen. I am unfamiliar with any comparisons of fenoprofen with indomethacin in rheumatoid arthritis but one early trial of ketoprofen compared 100 mg daily with 100 mg indomethacin in this disease (Gyory et al., 1972). The two drugs were similar in effect except when recourse to the rescue analgesic – in this case paracetamol – was measured. Significantly more paracetamol was needed by the ketoprofen patients than by those on indomethacin and this was again found in a further trial of 51 patients treated on a double-blind basis (Zutshi et al., 1974). Despite increasing the ketoprofen dose to 150 mg, leaving that of indomethacin at 100 mg, pain relief was significantly less and recourse to paracetamol significantly more in the ketoprofen-treated patients. Thus, indomethacin is seen to be equal to or more potent than the alternative analgesic/anti-inflammatory agents currently available.

Before leaving short-term studies I should like to highlight one aspect of indomethacin therapy which I find of great interest, that is the relief of night pain and morning stiffness. In an early study of indomethacin suppositories Holt and Hawkins (1965) suggested that peak plasma levels were delayed in comparison with oral medication. At the same time a marked decrease in morning stiffness was found and it became generally accepted that indomethacin suppositories were effective in the treatment of morning stiffness because of delay in absorption from the rectal mucosa. Subsequent work by Huskisson and his colleagues (1970) showed that the same dose given as capsules was if anything more effective than 100 mg in suppository form and a later study showed its superiority over both placebo and long-acting salicylate (Huskisson and Hart, 1972). Surprisingly it was discovered that night pain was a frequent reason for the prescription of barbiturates by British general practitioners so a further study compared the efficacy of indomethacin and amylobarbitone in relieving night pain and morning stiffness (Huskisson and Grayson, 1974). Indomethacin was rapidly shown to be significantly better and consequently proved more effective than the hypnotic in producing sleep in patients with rheumatoid arthritis. Barbiturates are less widely used now than in the past and I have for many years used diazepam at night in my patients, hoping that the sedative and anxiolytic properties might allow them to sleep and the muscle relaxant properties might decrease their morning stiffness. It therefore seemed appropriate to compare this non-barbiturate hypnotic with indomethacin at night and we have completed a trial of 10 mg diazepam versus 100 mg indomethacin versus placebo in in-patients with rheumatoid arthritis (Bayley and Haslock, 1976). Indomethacin was the most effective in reducing pain, though we were surprised to discover that diazepam was significantly better than placebo in this respect. Indomethacin also proved to be the best at producing sleep, although the differences were small. The effect on morning stiffness surprised us. Indomethacin again proved the best, but diazepam came out statistically significantly worse than placebo in this respect. We are at present conducting further experiments to try and find the reason for this. One other interesting fact that emerged was that there was no difference in side effects among the three therapeutic regimes over the short period of the trial.

As I mentioned earlier, rheumatoid arthritis is a long-term disease and long-term treatment is necessary. Long-term studies of indomethacin, in common with those of other drugs, are less rigorously controlled than short-term trials. Although in theory it would be possible to run groups of patients taking two or more types of treatment in parallel, in practice long-term studies tend to report the effect of treatment either in completely subjective terms or by use of sequential measurements or some manipulation of treatment in an attempt to quantify the drug's effectiveness. This means that the results must be interpreted with great caution, especially as rheumatoid arthritis is characterised by a fluctuating natural history. Despite these reservations, long-term studies deserve our careful attention because they are the nearest to our everyday clinic practice. They are also uniquely able to provide some types of information, such as the discovery by Smith (1965) in his 32-month study that the maximum anti-inflammatory effect of indomethacin did not occur until 2–4 months' treatment had elapsed in some of his patients. Arlet and Pujol (1966) were able to maintain 19 of 25 patients on indomethacin for up to 2 years in their study. They also found that they could reduce the dose while maintaining clinical effectiveness in one-third. In contrast, Thompson and Percy (1966) were able to continue treatment in only 44% of the 67 patients they studied for up to 82 weeks. Much larger numbers were used by Frankl (1966) who followed 441 patients with rheumatoid arthritis over a period of 20 months. He attempted to control his observations by discontinuing treatment in some patients, but found that indomethacin had to be rapidly re-introduced. Finally, I must pay tribute to the study of 757 patients reported by Bröll and his co-workers in 1972. They had studied patients continuously since indomethacin was introduced into their clinic in 1965. Of their 727 rheumatoid arthritis patients, 75 had stopped therapy because of side effects, all in the first month of treatment. They evaluated the remaining 658 patients as showing very good results in 29%, good results in 65% and moderate disease control only, requiring the use of additional drugs, in 6%. This study has now continued to contain over 1000 patients (Bröll, *This Volume*) and similar results still apply.

Laboratory testing in these studies did not reveal any significant long-term toxicity. This appears to be the general conclusion of laboratory testing, but clinical toxicity is a greater problem. The troublesome side effects of indomethacin lie in two main areas – gastrointestinal upset and CNS disturbance, especially headache. The long-term studies are almost unanimous regarding two things. First, the vast majority of side effects are seen during the first few weeks of therapy, few significant problems occurring in patients who tolerate this period of treatment. This does mean that indomethacin shows at its worst as regards side effects in short-term studies. Secondly, there is a need for individual dose adjustment. This has been demonstrated in the trials, and is obviously an integral part of good clinical practice. For example, my own upper limit of indomethacin dosage in rheumatoid arthritis is 50 mg 3 times daily plus 100 mg at night. I would obviously not use this 250-mg daily dose as starting therapy in rheumatoid arthritis, though I must add I would start patients with acute gout on much higher doses. One further point appears clear both from my own experience and from that of others which I have reviewed. The use of a large dose of indomethacin at night appears to be both effective and safe.

In summary it can be seen that indomethacin compares favourably with both new and established alternatives in the treatment of rheumatoid arthritis, that it is extremely effective in the management of night pain and morning stiffness and that side effects can be minimised by tailoring the dose of the drug to the individual patient.

References

ARLET, J. and PUJOL, M. (1966): Essai de traitement continu par l'indométacine des rheumatismes inflammatoires chroniques. *Sem. Hôp. Paris*, 42, 1727.

BAYLEY, T. R. L. and HASLOCK, I. (1976): Night medication in rheumatoid arthritis. *J. roy Coll. gen. Practit.*, in press.

BRÖLL, H., EBERL, R., SOCHAR, H. and TAUSCH, G. (1972): Verträglichkeit der langzeittherapie mit Indomethacin. *Wien. klin. Wschr.*, 84, 421.

CO-OPERATING CLINICS COMMITTEE OF THE AMERICAN RHEUMATISM ASSOCIATION (1967): A three-month trial of indomethacin in rheumatoid arthritis, with special reference to analysis and inference. *Clin. Pharmacol. Ther.*, 8, 11.

DICK, W. C., GRAYSON, M. F., WOODBURN, A., NUKI, G. and BUCHANAN, W. W. (1970): Indices of inflammatory activity. *Ann. rheum. Dis.*, *29*, 643.

D'OMÉZON, Y. (1973): Etude des cliniciens françois sur l'action de Naproxène dans la P.C.E. *Scand. J. Rheumatol.*, *Suppl. 2*, 164.

FRANKL, R. (1966): Long term treatment of chronic joint disorders (osteoarthritis, ankylosing spondylitis, gout) with particular reference to rheumatoid arthritis. In: *International Symposium on Inflammation, Freiburg im Breisgau*. Editors: R. Heister and H. F. Hofman. Urban and Schwarzenberg, Munich.

GYORY, A. N., BLOCK, M., BURRY, H. C. and GRAHAME, R. (1972): Orudis in management of rheumatoid arthritis and osteoarthrosis of the hip: comparison with indomethacin. *Brit. med. J.*, *4*, 398.

HART, F. D. and BOARDMAN, P. L. (1963): Indomethacin; a non-steroid anti-inflammatory agent. *Brit. med. J.*, *2*, 965.

HASLOCK, I., BURKINSHAW, L., BERRY, D., DONOVAN, B. and WRIGHT, V. (1976): Some studies of feprazone. *Rheumatol. and Rehab.*, *15*, 81.

HASLOCK, I., OMAR, A. S. and WRIGHT, V. (1975): A comparison of micro-encapsulated aspirin and indomethacin in the treatment of rheumatoid arthritis. *Brit. J. clin. Pract.*, *29*, 311.

HASLOCK, D. I., RHYMER, A. R., CHRISTIE, G. A. and WRIGHT, V. (1973): A comparative trial of naproxen and high dose indomethacin in rheumatoid arthritis – preliminary results. In: *Naprosyn in the treatment of Rheumatic Diseases – Proceedings of a Symposium, London;* Syntex, p. 35.

HERNANDEZ, L. A., McLEOD, M., GRENNAN, D. M., PALMER, D. G. and BUCHANAN, W. W. (1975): Clinical evaluation of two daily doses of naproxen and indomethacin: result of a double blind cross-over trial. *Curr. med. Res. and Opinion*, *3*, 359.

HOLT, L. P. J. and HAWKINS, C. F. (1965): Indomethacin: studies of absorption and of the use of indomethacin suppositories. *Brit. med. J.*, *1*, 1354.

HUSKISSON, E. C. and GRAYSON, M. F. (1974): Indomethacin or amylobarbitone sodium for sleep in rheumatoid arthritis, with some observations on the use of sequential analysis. *Brit. J. clin. Pharmacol.*, *1*, 151.

HUSKISSON, E. C. and HART, F. D. (1972): The use of indomethacin and aloxiprin at night. *Practitioner*, *208*, 248.

HUSKISSON, E. C., TAYLOR, R. T., BURSTON, D., CHUTER, P. J. and HART, F. D. (1970): Evening indomethacin in the treatment of rheumatoid arthritis. *Ann. rheum. Dis.*, *29*, 293.

JEREMY, R. and TOWSON, J. (1970): Interactions between aspirin and indomethacin in the treatment of rheumatoid arthritis. *Med. J. Austr.*, *2*, 127.

KOGSTAD, O. (1973): A double blind cross-over study of naproxen and indomethacin in patients with rheumatoid arthritis. *Scand. J. Rheumatol.*, *Suppl. 2*, 159.

LANSBURY, J. (1956): Quantitation of the activity of rheumatoid arthritis. V. A method for summation of the systemic indices of rheumatoid activity. *Amer. J. med. Sci.*, *232*, 300.

McGUIRE, R. F. and WRIGHT, V. (1971): Statistical approach to indices of disease activity in rheumatoid arthritis. *Ann. rheum. Dis.*, *30*, 574.

PITKEATHLY, D. A., BANERJEE, N. R., HARRIS, R. and SHARP, J. (1966): Indomethacin in inpatient treatment of rheumatoid arthritis. *Ann. rheum. Dis.*, *25*, 334.

RUBIN, A., RODDA, B. E., WARRICK, P., GRUBER, C. M. and RIDOLFO, A. S. (1973): Interactions of aspirin with non-steroidal anti-inflammatory drugs in man. *Arthr. Rheum.*, *16*, 635.

SMITH, C. J. (1965): Indomethacin in rheumatoid arthritis. A comparative objective evaluation with adrenocorticosteroids. *Arthr. Rheum.*, *8*, 921.

SZANTO, E. (1974): A doubleblind comparison of naproxen and indomethacin in rheumatoid arthritis. *Scand. J. Rheumatol.*, *3*, 118.

THOMPSON, M. and PERCY, J. S. (1966): Further experience with indomethacin in the treatment of rheumatic disorders. *Brit. med. J.*, *1*, 80.

WRIGHT, V., WALKER, W. C. and McGUIRE, R. J. (1969): Indomethacin in the treatment of rheumatoid arthritis. *Ann. rheum. Dis.*, *28*, 157.

ZUTSHI, D. W., STERN, D., BLOCK, M. and MASON, R. M. (1974): Ketoprofen: double blind cross-over study with indomethacin in patients with rheumatoid arthritis. *Rheumatol. and Rehab.*, *13*, 10.

The use of indomethacin in several febrile states. Ten years' experience

R. Marcolongo

Servizio di Reumatologia, University of Siena, Italy

Fever, which may be defined as any abnormal elevation in body temperature, is still considered an important and fascinating problem either from a theoretical point of view or as far as the therapeutical measures are concerned of preventing or controlling it. Some years ago indomethacin, a highly effective anti-inflammatory and analgesic drug, was reported to possess significant antipyretic action in experimental investigations (Benzi and Frigo, 1964; Winter et al., 1963), as well as in clinical studies (Ballabio et al., 1964; Hart and Boardman, 1964; Lusch et al., 1968; Marcolongo, 1971; Marcolongo et al., 1970; Marcolongo and Boggiano, 1966; Silberman et al., 1965; Treske, 1968; Winter et al., 1963). Experimental research has shown that indomethacin was more potent than aminopyrine, aspirin or phenylbutazone in preventing fever produced by injection of a bacterial lipopolysaccharide, in both rabbits and rats (Winter et al., 1963) (Fig. 1). A comparison of the more recent non-steroidal anti-inflammatory agents has proved that, at the minimum dose, the most effective antipyretic action on yeast fever in rats is that provided by indomethacin and diclofenac, as opposed to flufenamic acid, ibuprofen, phenylbutazone, naproxen and aspirin (Menassé, 1975) (Fig. 2). In clinical trials, indomethacin was found to bring about decrease of temperature in a wide variety of pyrexial disorders, both in adults and children, where other antipyretics have shown to be ineffective (Ballabio et al., 1964; Brewer, 1968; Giardini and Cardi, 1969; Hart and Boardman, 1964; Lusch et al., 1968; Marcolongo, 1971; Marcolongo et al., 1970;

°C
1.5
1
0.5
0
Increase in temperature above basal values
Controls
Phenylbutazone
Aminopyrine
Aspirin
Indomethacin
1
2
3
4
5
6
hr
Hours after injection of pyrogen

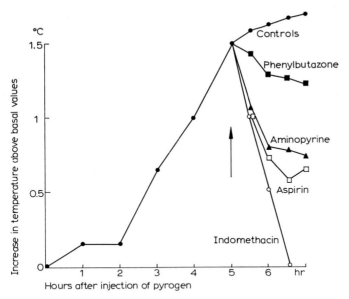

Fig. 1. Antipyretic effect of drugs orally administered to rats after temperature elevation by injection of a bacterial lipopolysaccharide. (From Winter et al., 1963; modified.)

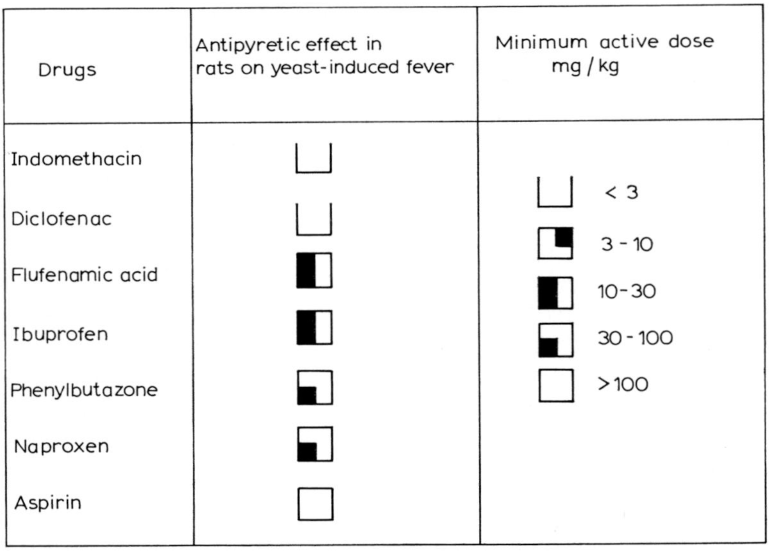

Drugs
Antipyretic effect in rats on yeast-induced fever
Minimum active dose mg / kg
Indomethacin
Diclofenac
Flufenamic acid
Ibuprofen
Phenylbutazone
Naproxen
Aspirin
< 3
3 - 10
10-30
30 - 100
>100

Fig. 2. Comparison of the antipyretic effect, at the minimum dose, of the more recent non-steroidal, anti-inflammatory drugs on fever induced in rats by yeast. (From Menassé, 1975; modified.)

Marcolongo and Boggiano, 1966; Marcolongo and DiPaolo, 1971; Silberman et al., 1965; Simila and Koivisto, 1968; Treske, 1968; Walker et al., 1966; Winter et al., 1963).

This paper concerns a number of experiments carried out to determine the antipyretic effectiveness of indomethacin in some febrile conditions, and further evaluate the possible mechanism of action of the drug.

Materials and methods

The first study was carried out on a group of 60 hospitalized patients with systemic hemopathies (15 with Hodgkin's disease, 15 with chronic lymphatic leukemia, 10 with chronic myeloid leukemia, 8 with acute myeloid leukemia, 5 with multiple myeloma, 1 with acute erythroleukemia, 2 with lymphosarcoma, and 4 with aplastic anemia), and 10 patients with malignant neoplasias (sigma, rectum, thyroid, lung, etc.), in whom fever was present and persisted despite therapy with cytotoxic agents, corticosteroids or the usual antipyretics. In those subjects in which fever cannot be attributed to bacterial or viral infections, treatment with indomethacin was initiated at doses of 25 mg orally every 6 hours, taking rectal temperature every 4 hours. The second experiment was carried out on 8 patients with severe tetanus and hyperpyrexia, to whom 200 mg/daily indomethacin was administered as suppositories. The third part of the study concerned 3 patients (aged 15–17) with juvenile rheumatoid arthritis (JRA) and hyperpyrexia resistant to corticosteroids and salicylates, to whom indomethacin was administered in doses of 75–100 mg daily. The final phase of the study was conducted as an evaluation of the efficacy of temperature control achieved by indomethacin in 30 healthy volunteers whose fever was induced by the administration of one intravenous injection of typhoid vaccine every 4 days for a total of four injections, at the same time controlling the antibody production rate. Fifteen of the subjects were given 100 mg/daily of indomethacin each day from the beginning of the experiment. The rectal temperature of all the subjects was taken every 4 hours.

Results

Indomethacin produced a significant antipyretic effect in all patients with Hodgkin's disease (Fig. 3), multiple myeloma, lymphosarcoma and aplastic anemia, within a few hours after receiving the drug. In patients with chronic lymphatic (Fig. 4) or myeloid leukemia the results were satisfactory, as a com-

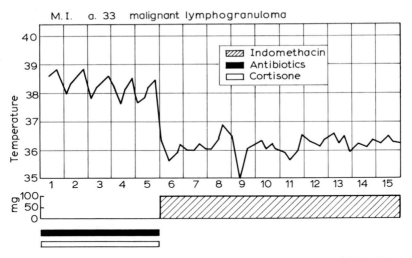

Fig. 3. Temperature response to indomethacin in a patient with Hodgkin's disease.

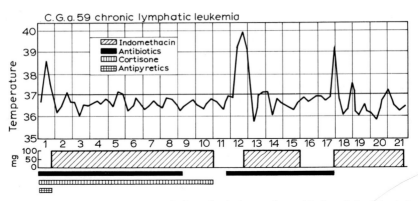

Fig. 4. Temperature response to indomethacin in a patient with chronic lymphatic leukemia.

plete defervescence occurred respectively in 66.6 and 50% of the cases. In subjects with myeloid acute leukemia and erythroleukemia, the antipyretic action
was evident in only 2 subjects out of 9 (22.2%). A significant antipyresis was
achieved in patients with malignant neoplasias: a complete defervescence occurred in 8 subjects (80%), while a moderate pyrexia persisted in the other 2
(Figs. 5 and 6). In all patients who responded to the treatment, a temperature
fall was detectable within a few hours after drug administration (in some cases
2–4 hours) or, at the most, within 24 hours. The patients reported symptomatic
improvement with marked regression of asthenia and general discomfort, which
continued during the period of indomethacin therapy and in some instances

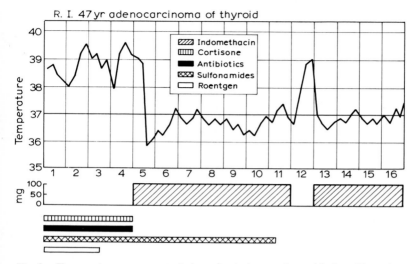

Fig. 5. Temperature response to indomethacin in a patient with thyroid carcinoma.

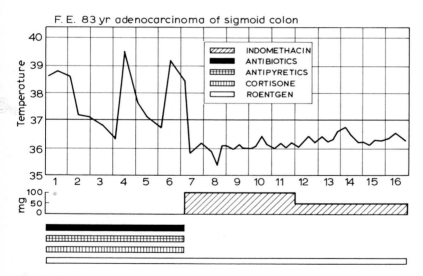

Fig. 6. Temperature response to indomethacin in a patient with sigmoid carcinoma.

could be maintained for as long as several months. The antipyretic effect persisted during the entire period of drug administration; when indomethacin was omitted, fever and subjective symptomatology promptly recurred, but again disappeared with re-institution of therapy (Fig. 7). In other subjects, in spite of suspension of treatment, the defervescence persisted for variable periods of

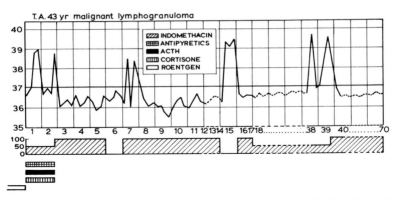

Fig. 7. Temperature response to indomethacin in a patient with Hodgkin's disease. Fever controlled by drug treatment relapsed rapidly with cessation of the therapy. Resumption of indomethacin again resulted in a prompt control of pyrexia.

time. Drug resistance was not observed. We emphasize that a full dose of the drug, usually from 75–100 mg/daily, must be administered to achieve the anti-pyretic effect. Some patients initially treated with too low doses showed either an incomplete remission or a rapid reappearance of fever. In addition, it is well known that indomethacin is adsorbed to a high degree from the gastrointestinal tract rather promptly after oral administration, and peak plasma levels appear within 60–90 minutes, reaching the lowest levels at 6–8 hours (Caruso et al., 1964; Hart and Boardman, 1964). It is therefore evident that the drug must be given in divided doses during the day, 6 hours appearing to be the maximum interval to maintain adequate plasma concentrations (Marcolongo, 1971; Silberman et al., 1965).

Indomethacin did not show significant results in any of the 8 patients with severe tetanus and hyperpyrexia, and fever was not at all influenced by the ad-ministration of the drug (Fig. 8). Four of the patients died with a marked hyperpyrexia, while in the other cases the fever fell as the clinical conditions of the patients improved, to disappear completely when they were in convales-cence. In the 3 patients with JRA, the response to indomethacin treatment was excellent, with a rapid, dramatic fall and disappearance of fever in a few hours and a subsequent complete control of the temperature (Fig. 9). In the 15 sub-jects who were given typhoid vaccine without indomethacin treatment, the temperature rose significantly from 6–16 hours after vaccine injection (Fig. 10). Fever continued for from 18–42 hours, with temperatures between 38.2°C and 39.8°C, accompanied by chills, severe headache and general malaise. The anti-body response was good: 12 days after the first vaccine injection, all subjects showed high antibody levels against both O and H antigens (Fig. 11). The other

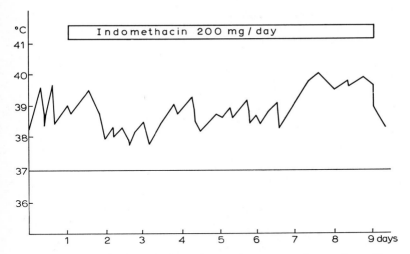

Fig. 8. Inability of indomethacin to decrease temperature in a patient with severe tetanus and hyperpyrexia.

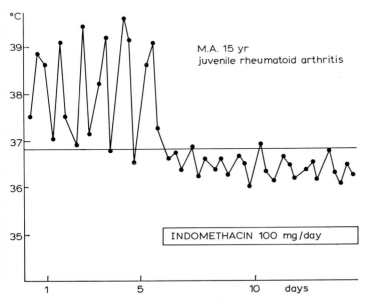

Fig. 9. Temperature response to indomethacin in a patient with juvenile rheumatoid arthritis.

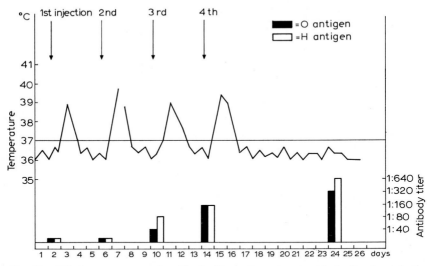

Fig. 10. Febrile responses and antibody titers of a normal subject after i.v. injections of typhoid vaccine.

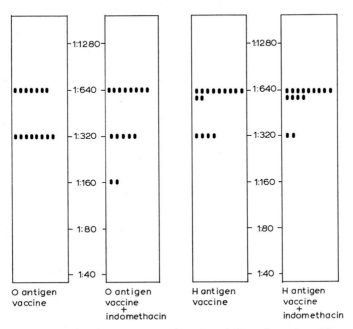

Fig. 11. Antibody response against O and H antigens in subjects treated with typhoid vaccine or with vaccine and indomethacin.

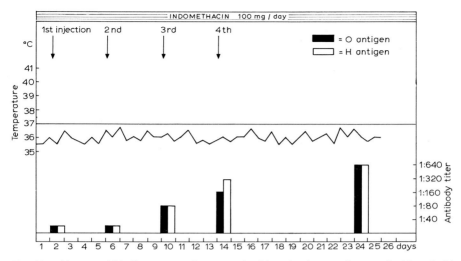

Fig. 12.   Absence of febrile responses in a normal subject simultaneously treated with typhoid vaccine and indomethacin.

15 subjects treated with typhoid vaccine and at the same time with indomethacin, did not show any rise in temperature, which remained within normal values (Fig. 12). Only in 2 cases, where after the 2nd vaccine dose indomethacin was erroneously not given for 24 hours, hyperpyrexia appeared which, however, promptly disappeared upon immediate resumption of the drug (Fig. 13). The antibody response in the indomethacin-treated subjects was identical to that of the former group. Furthermore, none of them suffered from accompanying subjective symptomatology and the vaccination was practically unperceived by these subjects. At the administered dose schedule, no untoward reactions were observed in any patient of the various groups studied.

Discussion

The interpretation of the mode of action of indomethacin in producing its antipyretic effect is still unknown. It is well established that this action does not depend upon stimulation of the pituitary-adrenal axis (Ballabio et al., 1964; Winter et al., 1963). A possible mechanism might be a peripheral influence of the drug on the formation and/or the release of endogenous pyrogen by the leukocytes. Though there has been intensive investigation on the physiological mechanisms which regulate body temperature, the pathogenesis of fever has remained obscure for many years. Recent knowledge on the pathogenesis of

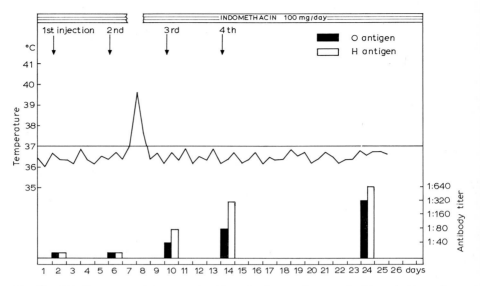

Fig. 13. Febrile response in a normal subject simultaneously treated with typhoid vaccine and indomethacin. The omission of indomethacin for 24 hours after the 2nd vaccine dose esulted in hyperpyrexia, which promptly disappeared upon immediate re-institution of the antipyretic therapy.

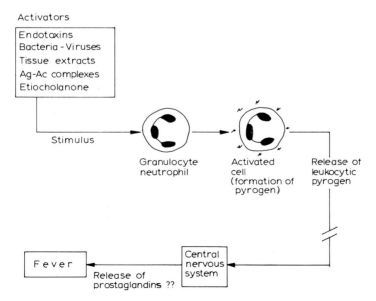

Fig. 14. Postulated pathways in the pathogenesis of fever.

fever support the view that most fevers are caused by action on the hypothalamic region of the central nervous system of an endogenous pyrogen (EP) produced and released from polymorphonuclear leukocytes, when these cells are *activated* by a variety of both microbial and non-microbial stimuli (endotoxins, bacteria, viruses, antigen-antibody complexes, tissue extracts) (Atkins and Bodel, 1972; Cooper, 1966; Editorial, 1967; Petersdorf, 1968) (Fig. 14). However, the frequent occurrence of high fevers in diseases such as agranulocytosis and acute monocytic leukemia suggested that cells other than granulocytes release EP: experimental observations provided good evidence that EP can be also produced by monocytes and macrophages (Atkins and Bodel, 1972; Editorial, 1967). The recent findings on defervescence after treatment with salicylates lead to the conclusion that the antipyretic action is not due to a peripheral action on the leukocytes by preventing the formation and release of EP or by destroying EP before it reaches the brain, but can be attributed to their direct action on the hypothalamic thermoregulatory centers (Adler et al., 1969; Gander et al., 1967; Hoo et al., 1972). Also in the case of indomethacin the hypothesis has been made that the antipyretic effect might be mediated by a direct action on the hypothalamus. This hypothesis is supported by the observation of 3 patients with cerebral hemorrhage and hyperpyrexia related to disturbances of thermoregulatory centers, in whom temperature fell within a few hours after administration of indomethacin suppositories (Marcolongo and Boggiano, 1966). From a theoretical point of view, the best condition for verifying a possible central action of indomethacin seemed to be the series of patients with severe tetanus and hyperpyrexia. However, the results obtained were negative and inconclusive to elucidate the mechanism by which the drug produces its antipyretic effect. It must, however, be emphasized that in addition to diseases in which fever is mediated by an EP release from activated leukocytes, there are some conditions in which EP probably has no role in producing elevated temperature. In tetanus, it seems likely that indomethacin is on one hand unable to act on the impaired hypothalamic thermoregulatory centers, and on the other unable to bring the hypothalamic *thermostat* to normal values, because of the continuous heat production originating in the periphery, due to the marked muscular rigidity and repeated spasms (Adams et al., 1969). The problem, however, is complicated by the observation that fever was produced in man by injection of etiocholanone (3α-hydroxy-5β-androstan-17-one), a naturally occurring metabolite of androgenic hormones (Bodel et al., 1968; Bondy et al., 1965; Wolff et al., 1973) and by the presence of increased plasma concentrations of etiocholanone reported in some patients with neoplasias, Hodgkin's disease, and other febrile diseases (George et al., 1969; Wolff et al., 1973). Although the mechanism by which this hormone metabolite produces fever is unknown, it

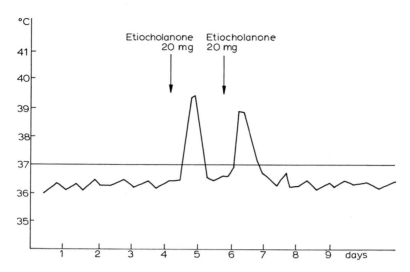

Fig. 15. Typical febrile response in a normal subject after 2 successive intramuscular injections of etiocholanone.

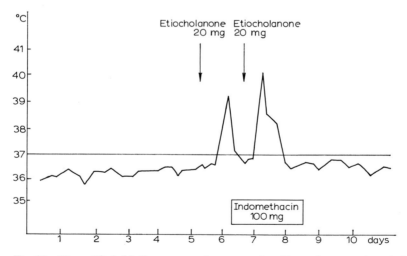

Fig. 16. Unmodified febrile response in a normal subject who was given indomethacin simultaneously with the second injection of etiocholanone.

seems likely that the local inflammatory reaction at the site of injection is essential to its pyrogenicity (Wolff et al., 1973).

We carried out some experiments on this subject (Marcolongo, 1971). Etiocholanone (Sigma Chemical Co., St. Louis, U.S.A.) prepared in propylene

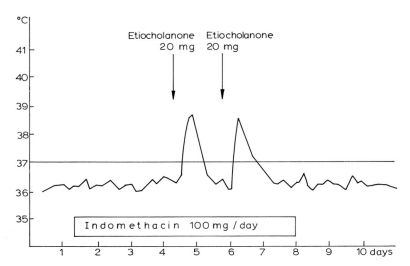

Fig. 17. Unmodified febrile response in a normal subject who was given indomethacin for 3 successive days before the first etiocholanone injection.

glycol, 10 mg/ml was administered at 8 a.m. to 10 male healthy volunteers (aged 25–44), at a dosage of 20 mg; the injection was repeated the next day, taking rectal temperature at 4-hour intervals for 24 hours after injections (Fig. 15). Indomethacin was administered orally at a dose of 100 mg/daily, simultaneously with the second injection of etiocholanone and then continued (Fig. 16), cr was administered for 3 successive days before the first hormone injection and then continued (Fig. 17). The results of these experiments, however, were inconclusive to explain the absence of the antipyretic effect of indomethacin, and of scarce value in elucidating the mechanism of action of the drug.

Although the biochemical basis for the indomethacin action is not clear, the more likely hypothesis suggests that this drug might influence some step of the temperature-regulating system through the following mechanisms (Fig. 18): (1) peripheral action on leukocytes (or other cells) by preventing the formation and/or release of endogenous cellular pyrogens; (2) inactivation of cellular pyrogens before they can reach the central nervous system; (3) direct action on the hypothalamic thermoregulatory centers. A fourth mechanism is, however, possible. Recently, a new area of investigation into the cause of fever has been opened up by the observation that certain prostaglandins (PGs), that are present in the brain as well as in other tissues, are reported to be pyrogenic when injected into the hypothalamus of laboratory animals, so suggesting that PGs could be a molecular transmitter of pyrogenic stimuli in the hypothalamic centers (Atkins and Bodel, 1972; Milton and Wendlandt, 1971). Consequently,

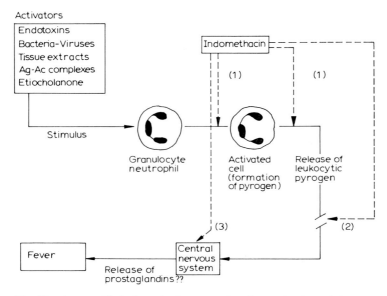

Fig. 18. A more likely hypothesis concerning the mcehanism of the antipyretic action of indomethacin (see text).

it has been suggested that the antipyretic action of aspirin may be related to the inhibition of synthesis of pyrogenic PGs (Atkins and Bodel, 1972). Although the capacity for indomethacin to inhibit PG activities seems well established (Flower, 1974; Vane, 1971), further work is needed to define if this is the physiological mechanism of the antipyretic action of the drug in man.

In any case, indomethacin has proved to possess a significant antipyretic effect which can be usefully utilized in the symptomatic treatment of fever in Hodgkin's disease, multiple myeloma, chronic lymphatic and myeloid leukemia and malignant neoplasias. The suppression of the subjective symptomatology directly attributable to fever (malaise, asthenia, chills, and anorexia), efficiently integrates the action of corticosteroids, or chemotherapy. Indomethacin showed the greatest antipyretic effect in patients with a very high temperature or fever resistant to other antipyretic drugs, and in those subjects whose clinical conditions require a highly effective antipyretic agent. The antipyretic treatment should, however, be initiated only after a complete evaluation of the clinical picture, exclusion of infective complications and an adequate cycle of chemotherapy, keeping in mind that defervescence does not exclude the possibility of an underlying infection (Marcolongo, 1971; Silberman et al., 1965). Non-steroidal anti-inflammatory drugs must always be considered from the point of view of a possible facilitating or masking effect of an infectious process. Contrary to corticosteroids (Marcolongo, 1971; Marcolongo and DiPaolo, 1971), indomethacin did not decrease resistance to infections in laboratory animals, even if given in large doses (Manganaro and Baldasserini, 1969; Merck, Sharp and Dohme, 1964). On the other hand, it has never been shown that this drug favors the onset of secondary infections in man or produces immunological disturbances, even if some authors suggested that indomethacin could decrease the host's response to infections, reactivating latent infections (Rodriguez and Barbabosa, 1971; Solomon, 1966).

On the basis of our results, the association of indomethacin treatment in subjects actively immunized with vaccines seems to be particularly interesting in relation to the possibility of utilizing its anti-inflammatory and antipyretic properties to avoid the side effects appearing during the vaccination, without influencing the antibody response. The utility of a more widespread utilization of this treatment in association with other types of vaccine would thus seem evident, as well as investigations to ascertain whether the same excellent results obtained in adults can also be obtained in children. Although indomethacin has not been recommended in pediatric patients because of some reports of sudden death or hepatitis (Jacobs, 1967; Kelsey and Sharys, 1967), many authors have studied the effectiveness of this drug to control fever, as compared to other antipyretics, without apparently any serious complications (Brewer, 1968; Giardini and Cardi, 1969; Simila and Koivosto, 1968; Walker et al., 1966). Indomethacin seems also to be indicated in patients with JRA, which often show serious subjective symptomatology and hyperpyrexia which could not be controlled despite therapy with common antipyretics, or even corticosteroids.

In conclusion, on the basis of our experience over a period of 10 years, we can affirm that the tolerance and the absence of untoward effects, and the marked antipyretic potency of indomethacin in a wide variety of diseases, represent a very interesting clinical finding and a certain advantage when compared with the common antipyretic drugs usually utilized in the symptomatic treatment of fever present in some physiological and pathological states.

References

ADAMS, E. B., LAURENCE, D. R. and SMITH, J. W. G. (1969): *Tetanus*. Blackwell, Oxford.

ADLER, R. D., RAWLINS, M., ROSENDORFF, C. and CRANSTON, W. I. (1969): The effect of salicylate on pyrogen-induced fever in man. *Clin. Sci.*, *37*, 91.

ATKINS, E. and BODEL, P. (1972): Fever. *New Engl. J. Med.*, *286*, 27.

BALLABIO, C. B., GRASSI, F., RIMOLDI, R. and FEDRIGA, G. (1964): Indicazioni extrareumatologiche dell'Indometacin. *Atti Accad. med. lombarda, 19*, 37.

BENZI, G. and FRIGO, G. M. (1964): Ipertermia da pirogeni batterici nel ratto e sua utilizzazione nel saggio dell'attività antipiretica. *Il Farmaco, 19*, 498.

BODEL, P. T., DILLARD, M. and BONDY, P. K. (1968): The mechanism of steroid-induced fever. *Ann. intern. Med., 69*, 875.

BONDY, P. K., COHN, G. L. and GREGORY, P. B. (1965): Etiocholanolone fever. *Medicine (Baltimore), 44*, 249.

BREWER, E. J. (1968): A comparative evaluation of Indomethacin, Acetaminophen, and Placebo as antipyretic agents in children. *Arthr. and Rheum., 11*, 645.

CARUSO, I., FORCELLA, E. and MARCAZZAN, E. (1964): Il comportamento del tasso plasmatico dell'indometacin. *Reumatismo, 16*, 393.

COOPER, K. E. (1966): Temperature regulation and the hypothalamus. *Brit. med. Bull., 22*, 2.

EDITORIAL (1967): Pathogenesis of fever. *New Engl. J. Med., 276*, 1036.

FLOWER, R. J. (1974): Drugs which inhibit prostaglandin biosynthesis. *Pharmacol. Rev., 26*, 33.

GANDER, G. W., CHAFFEE, J. and GOODALE, F. (1967): Studies on the antipyretic action of salicylates. *Proc. Soc. exp. Biol. (N.Y.), 126*, 205.

GEORGE, J. M., WOLFF, S. M., DILLER, E. and BARTTER, F. C. (1969): Recurrent fever of unknown etiology; failure to demonstrate association between fever and plasma unconjugated etiocholanolone. *J. clin. Invest., 48*, 558.

GIARDINI, O. and CARDI, E. (1969): Studio clinico sull'azione antipiretica dell'indometacina nell'infanzia. *Policlinico, Sez. med., 76*, 322.

HART, F. D. and BOARDMAN, P. L. (1964): Indomethacin. *Practitioner, 192*, 828.

HOO, S. L., LIN, M. T., WEI, R. D., CHAI, C. Y. and WAUG, S. C. (1972): Effects of sodium acetylsalicylate on the release of pyrogen from leukocytes. *Proc. Soc. exp. Biol. (N.Y.), 139*, 1155.

JACOBS, J. C. (1967): Sudden death in arthritic children receiving large doses of indomethacin. *J. Amer. med. Ass., 199*, 932.

KELSEY, W. M. and SHARYS, M. (1967): Fatal hepatitis probably due to indomethacin. *J. Amer. med. Ass., 199*, 586.

LUSCH, C. J., SERPICK, A. A. and SLATER, L. (1968): Antipyretic effect of Indomethacin in patients with malignancy. *Cancer, 21*, 781.

MANGANARO, M. and BALDASSERINI, G. (1969): Azione di alcuni anti-infiammatori non steroidei a paragone con quella del prednisone nel topo albino in corso di vaccinazione antitifo. *Boll. Soc. ital. Biol. sper., 45*, 851.

MARCOLONGO, R. (1971): L'effetto antipiretico dell'Indometacina in alcune condizioni morbose. *Atti Simp. Int. Infiammazione e sua Terapia, Firenze*, p. 385. Soc. Editrice Universo, Rome.

MARCOLONGO, R., BIANCO, G., DI PAOLO, N. and BRAVI, A. (1970): Ricerche cliniche sull'effetto antipiretico dell'Indometacin nelle emopatie sistemiche. *Minerva med., 61*, 4532.

MARCOLONGO, R. and BOGGIANO, C. A. (1966): Sull'azione antipiretica dell'Indometacin nel linfogranuloma di Hodgkin e nelle neoplasie. *Minerva med., 57*, 2857.

MARCOLONGO, R. and DIPAOLO, N. (1971): L'impiego dell'Indometacin in soggetti sottoposti a vaccinazione. *Boll. Ist. sieroter. milan., 50*, 409.

MENASSÉ, R. (1975): Metodi sperimentali per la caratterizzazione di farmaci antiflogistici. In: Simposio su: *Tollerabilità ed Efficacia nella Moderna Terapia Antireumatica Nonsteroidea, S. Margherita di Pula (Sardegna)*. Ciba–Geigy, Basle.

MERCK, SHARP and DOHME (1964): *Report on Indomethacin and infection.*

MILTON, A. S. and WENDLANDT, S. (1971): Effects on body temperature of prostaglandins of the A, E and F series on injection into the third ventricle of unanaesthetized cats and rabbits. *J. Physiol. (Lond.), 218*, 325.

PETERSDORF, R. G. (1968): The physiology, pathogenesis and diagnosis of fever. *Med. Times, 96*, 50.

RODRIGUEZ, R. and BARBABOSA, E. (1971): Hemorrhagic chicken pox after indomethacin. *New Engl. J. Med., 285*, 690.

SILBERMAN, H. R., McGINN, T. G. and KREMER, W. B. (1965): Control of fever in Hodgkin's disease by Indomethacin. *J. Amer. med. Ass., 194*, 598.

SIMILA, S. and KOIVISTO, M. (1968): Indomethacin as an antipyretic agent in pediatrics. *Clin. Pediat., 7*, 69.

SOLOMON, L. (1966): Activation of latent infection by Indomethacin: a report of three cases. *Brit. med. J., 1*, 961.

TRESKE, U. (1968): Indomethacin und Hämatopoese. Antipyretische und antiphlogistische Wirkung bei Hämoblastosen und einigen seltenen Krankheitsbildern. *Med. Klin., 63*, 344.

VANE, J. R. (1971): Inhibition of prostaglandin synthesis as a mechanism of action for aspirin-like drugs. *Nature New Biol., 231*, 232.

WALKER, S. H., HOFFMAN, S. H., SILVERSTONE, L. and DIMOIA, F. (1966): The antipyretic effect of Indomethacin: a clinical study of the use for fever states in man. *Clin. Pediat., 5*, 204.

WINTER, C. A., RISLEY, E. A. and NUSS, G. W. (1963): Anti-inflammatory and antipyretic activities of Indomethacin, 1-(p-chlorobenzoyl)-5-methoxy-2-methyl-indole-3-acetic acid. *J. Pharmacol. exp. Therap., 141*, 369.

WOLFF, S. M., KIMBALL, H. R. and MARSHALL, J. R. (1973): The effects of hydrocortisone and estrogen on experimental fever induced by etiocholanolone. *J. infect. Dis., 128*, 243.

Indomethacin in the management of soft tissue lesions

H. C. Burry

Guy's Arthritis Research Unit, Guy's Hospital Medical School, London, United Kingdom

In examining the role of indomethacin therapy in the management of soft tissue lesions, the author commences by examining the theoretical basis for its use by comparing the known pharmacological properties of indomethacin with the known pathology of soft tissue injury. Indomethacin has been shown to have the following properties (Table 1). Of these, granuloma inhibition, suppression of oedema, analgesic properties, prostaglandin synthetase inhibition and stabilisation of lysosomal membranes are features which might well prove useful in the management of soft tissue injury.

The pathology of soft tissue injury of traumatic origin is summarised in Table 2 and the complications which one wishes to counter with appropriate therapy

TABLE 1

Pharmacological properties of indomethacin

1. Granuloma inhibition
2. Oedema suppression in carrageenan test
3. Suppression of adjuvant arthritis
4. Mild analgesia
5. Inhibition of lymphocyte stimulation by PHA
6. Prostaglandin synthetase inhibition
7. ? Stabilisation of lysosomal membranes

TABLE 2

Pathology of soft tissue lesions

A. TRAUMATIC
   Rupture of tissue
   Extravasation of blood
   → Prostaglandin and kinins released
   → Vasodilation and oedema
   Repair by organisation of haematoma
   Fibrinolysis
   Endothelial proliferation
   Phagocytosis
   Fibroblastic proliferation
   Myoblastic proliferation

TABLE 3

Complications of soft tissue injury

1. Pain
2. Excessive oedema (causing limitation of muscle power and joint movement and muscle atrophy)
3. Inadequate repair
4. Adhesion
5. Organised haematoma
6. Massive fibrosis
7. Encysted haematoma
8. Calcification
9. Ossification

are shown in Table 3. Of these, pain, excessive oedema which leads to a limitation of muscle power and joint movement, and therefore to muscle atrophy, adhesions, formation of organised haematoma and possibly a massive fibrosis are features which might well be modified by treatment with a potent anti-inflammatory drug. In Table 4 are displayed the pathological features of such degenerative soft tissue lesions as enthesopathies, chronic tendinitis, tenosynovitis and periarthritis. In these granuloma formation, oedema and hyperaemia and possibly fibrosis and formation of adhesions are likely to be affected by anti-inflammatory drug therapy. To these conditions, perhaps there should be added acute and chronic spinal lesions such as prolapsed intervertebral disc with or without radicular involvement. In this situation the injury to the disc is

TABLE 4

Pathology of soft tissue lesions

DEGENERATIVE

1. ENTHESOPATHIES
   Degeneration of collagenous fibres and
   fibrocytes
   Granuloma formation
   Calcification
   Fibroblastic proliferation
   New collagen formation

2. CHRONIC TENDINITIS
   Degeneration of collagenous fibres
   Granuloma formation
   Fibroblastic proliferation
   New collagen formation
   Ossification (rarely)

3. TENOSYNOVITIS
   Reduplication of synovial lining cells
   Oedema and hyperaemia
   Adhesions

4. PERIARTHRITIS
   Oedema
   Hyperaemia
   Calcification
   Fibrosis
   Adhesions

accompanied by a brisk inflammatory reaction with hyperaemia, oedema and in some cases, formation of adhesions between the nerve root and the dura. Here again, indomethacin might well prove effective.

Clinical experience with indomethacin in soft tissue injury

Having shown a theoretical basis and rationalisation of the use of indomethacin in soft tissue injury, we can now examine the literature pertaining to this subject. Three 'open' studies should be mentioned initially. Von Baumann and Hoffman (1971) reported the use of indomethacin in a dose of 150–200 mg per day in acute or subacute rheumatism. They found impressive results, particularly in acute spinal lesions with radicular symptoms and found that the known central nervous system and gastrointestinal symptoms might be reduced greatly by using a combined oral and rectal route of administration enabling the bulk of the dosage to be given in the evening. Von Penners (1971) reported experience of some 800 children who had received indomethacin after orthopaedic surgery and felt that the good results obtained in terms of reduced pain and post-operative oedema justified the use of the drug routinely. Von Muller (1971) collected 240 cases of soft tissue rheumatism including periarthritis of the shoulder, lumbar back ache and bursitis. Good results were seen when indomethacin was used as an adjunct to physiotherapy and there were no serious side effects.

Controlled trials of indomethacin in soft tissue lesions

The literature contains 6 controlled trials of indomethacin. Of these, the work of Fitch and Gray (1974) and Huskisson et al. (1973) pertains to the use of indomethacin in sports injuries. Fitch and Gray reported significant improvement, but Huskisson et al. showed no benefits, probably because the proportion of cases who recovered was high in both the group treated with indomethacin and the control subjects.

When Van Marion (1973) studied 83 patients with traumatic soft tissue injuries, indomethacin was prescribed in a dose of between 100 and 150 mg and compared with placebo. All patients received also crepe bandaging of the injured part and rest. Double-blind conditions were preserved and on analysis of results, indomethacin at a dosage of 150 mg was found to be significantly superior to placebo in terms of relief of spontaneous pain and decreased tenderness, swelling and limitation of movement.

Jacobs and Hicklin (1963) compared indomethacin with placebo in the management of painful shoulder and in acute low back pain in a double-blind controlled trial. Their results showed that indomethacin was superior in the painful shoulder cases but they were unable to show a significant advantage in management of acute low back pain. In a further trial, Jacobs found indomethacin, 75 mg daily, to be significantly superior to placebo in a group of patients suffering from painful, stiff shoulders.

Scott and Wynne-Hughes (1967) reported the results of 2 double-blind trials. In the first, 45 patients were studied and oxyphenbutazone was compared with a placebo under double-blind conditions, while in the second, which included 35 patients, oxyphenbutazone was compared with indomethacin also under double-blind conditions. Their patients were suffering from low back pain, arthritic pain, fibrositis and structural lesions of the cervical spine. In these patients there was a trend in favour of oxyphenbutazone but statistical significance was not achieved. However, when the group of lesions of the cervical spine, which the authors considered were unlikely to respond to drug therapy without additional physical therapy, were excluded, a further analysis showed a statistically significant response. Oxyphenbutazone was then compared with indomethacin under double-blind conditions and the 2 drugs were found to produce almost identical results. Indomethacin, although causing approximately the same proportion of side effects as oxyphenbutazone, apparently produced more severe symptoms, in that 3 patients had to be withdrawn from treatment. No serious toxic effects were noted.

Conclusions

1. There are good theoretical reasons for expecting indomethacin to be effective in the management of soft tissue lesions.
2. Good results have been obtained in double-blind controlled trials comparing indomethacin with placebo and with oxyphenbutazone, confirming results seen in open trials.
3. Side effects have usually been minor, rarely causing patients to be withdrawn from treatment.
4. Nevertheless, the possibility of serious side effects such as peptic ulceration, blood dyscrasias, hypertension and fluid retention must be borne in mind when considering using indomethacin to treat conditions which are likely to resolve even without drug therapy.

References

FITCH, K. D. and GRAY, S. D. (1974): *Med. J. Aust.*, *1*, 260.
HUSKISSON, E. G. et al. (1973): *Rheumatol. and Rehab.*, *12*, 159.
SCOTT, R. S. and WYNNE-HUGHES, I. (1967): *J. Ther. clin. Res.*, *1*, 17.
VAN MARION, W. F. (1973): *J. int. med. Res.*, *1*, 151.
VON BAUMANN, J. C. and HOFFMANN, U. (1971): *Arzneimittel-Forsch.*, *11a*, 1875.
VON MULLER, G. (1971): *Arzneimittel-Forsch.*, *11a*, 1876.
VON PENNERS, R. (1971): *Arzneimittel-Forsch.*, *11a*, 1842.

The natural history of chronic rheumatic diseases of the joint and the value of surgery within general therapy

D. Wessinghage

Operative Klinik des Rheumazentrums, Bad Abbach/Regensburg, Federal Republic of Germany

Chronic rheumatic diseases of the joint manifest themselves through an inflammation of the synovial membrane of joints, but also in tendon sheaths and bursae. Prominent in the proliferative phase of rheumatoid arthritis, psoriatic arthritis and ankylosing spondylitis (with peripheral joint involvement) is the inflammatory hypertrophy and hyperplasia of the entire synovial lining of the joint (Fig. 1). A synovial pannus which starts from the osteochondral junction and grows over the hyaline cartilage is also an expression of the proliferative effect (Fig. 2). Under this pannus in particular, the destruction of the cartilage begins. Destruction occurs by reason of synovial tissue growing into bone and cartilage (destructive phase) so that finally the typical deformation of the joint can result. At the same time, the tissue mass, and also the increasing formation of tissue fluid and fibrin as products of inflammation, cause an over-extension of the joint capsule and the ligaments. The damage and destruction of the joint surfaces and the capsular ligamentous apparatus produce incongruity of the joint surfaces, and also instability of the joint. The consequence of this is a secondary arthrosis in the degenerative phase with corresponding damage to the cartilage and reparative changes in the form of development of a marginal ridge and chondro-osteophytes (Fig. 3).

If the inflammatory activity of rheumatoid arthritis returns to the degenerative phase, and a new inflammatory exacerbation can no longer be counted on, the burned out phase is reached. In this, proliferative and destructive changes no longer increase, while advancement of the secondary arthrosis is certainly possible (Fig. 4).

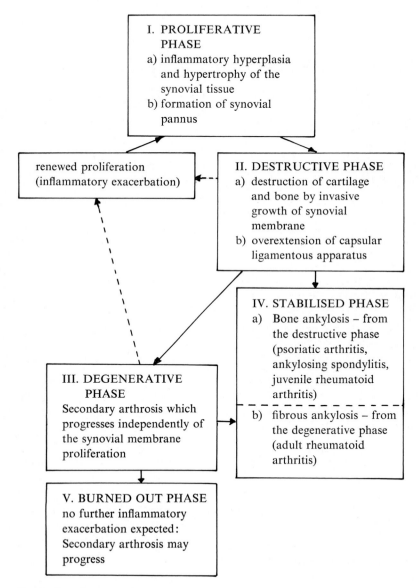

Fig. 1. Development of rheumatoid arthritis.

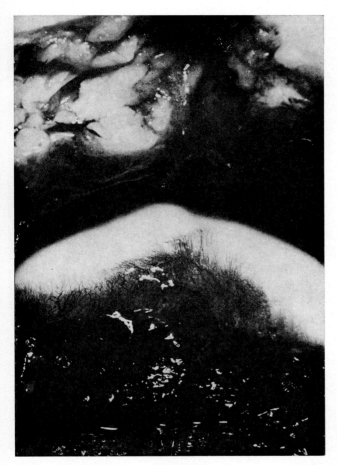

Fig. 2. Proliferation of synovial pannus growing over the hyaline cartilage.

In rheumatoid arthritis in adults, a fibrous ankylosis may develop from the degenerative phase (Fig. 5). Stabilisation occurs: in the affected joint both the function – it will be completely abolished – and the disease process are stabilised. The stiffening is followed by a regression of the synovial membrane so that the disease is deprived of its site of manifestation.

In different diseases of the joints, such as juvenile rheumatoid arthritis (Still's disease), psoriatic arthritis and ankylosing spondylitis, the destructive phase can pass directly into the stabilised phase.

While in the destructive and degenerative phases a fresh proliferative synovitis may appear with each exacerbation, this is no longer possible during the stabilised and the burned out phase.

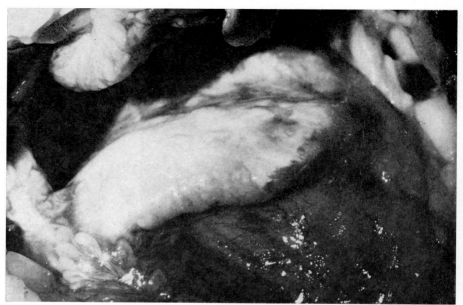

Fig. 3. Secondary arthrosis (osteoarthritis) in the degenerative phase with marginal ridge and damage to the cartilage. Active inflammation seen by proliferative formation of the synovial membrane.

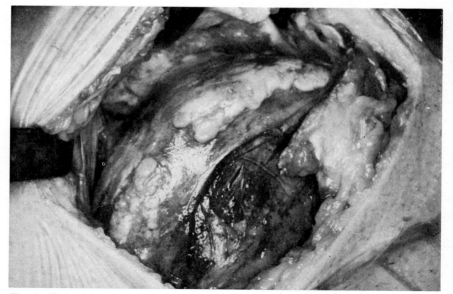

Fig. 4. Burned out case of rheumatoid arthritis without any inflammatory activity but with degenerative changes.

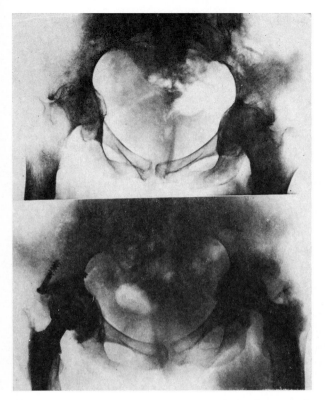

Fig. 5. Fibrous ankylosing of hip joints with development of protrusio acetabuli in an adult case of rheumatoid arthritis. Endoprostheses of the hip joints.

The medical treatment of rheumatoid arthritis is symptomatic by non-steroidal antirheumatics (indometacin, butazone derivatives, salicylates and others), and corticosteroids, basal therapeutics (chloroquine, gold salts, D-penicillamine, cytostatics) and surgical. Physiotherapy, balneological and general measures are used in support (Fig. 6).

In the operative treatment of rheumatic diseases of the joints, preventive and palliative or reconstructive operations are differentiated. Early synovectomy undertaken in the proliferative phase is very often able to prevent, or at least to stop, increasing joint damage. Quite often there is a considerable improvement in the symptoms and mobility, since destructive and degenerative changes do not yet exist. Relapses of synovitis are fortunately rare post-operatively. A general regression of the inflammatory activity of the disease is, of course, occasionally questioned, but we have been able to ascertain this as a

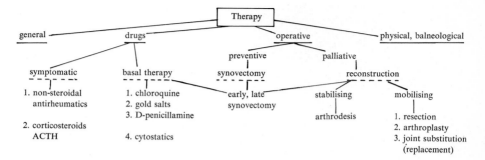

Fig. 6.   Therapeutic possibilities in rheumatoid arthritis.

result of numerous consecutive follow-up examinations after synovectomy of the knee joint. The regression of the titre seems to pave the way for a more favourable development of the rheumatoid factor postoperatively.

An objectifiable improvement in the findings can also be demonstrated in some of the patients by consecutive radiological examinations, even in a more advanced phase of the disease. Thus we were able to recognise an improvement in the osteoporosis around the joint, a regression of destructive changes and even a postoperative reforming of the cartilage, which has often largely disappeared – recognisable by the widening of the radiological interarticular space – with increasing movement and load.

In spite of good results after radioactive or chemical sclerosing of the synovial membrane, early synovectomy will not, in our opinion, lose its importance in the treatment of rheumatic patients.

In addition to late synovectomy, palliative or reconstructive interventions include other mobilising and stabilising operations. By late synovectomy, mechanical impairment of the joint function must be achieved by removal of synovial tissue masses, free arthrophytes, marginal ridges, and intra-articular lipoids. Moreover, stabilisation of incompetent ligaments and the elimination of contractures, among other things, are essential. Also, these measures cannot be superseded by so-called 'synoviorthesis'.

Unstable, deformed joints which are no longer capable of bearing a load and false positions must be treated by arthrodesis – that is, a stabilising operation. By elimination of the residual function of a joint, improvement in the entire function of the extremity can be attained. Neighbouring joints of the same or contralateral extremities may usually show no lesion. In rheumatic patients, arthrodeses are performed by different methods on knee, ankle, wrist and also on finger joints (Fig. 7).

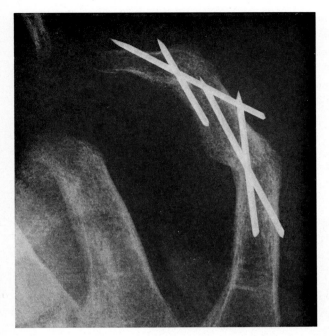

Fig. 7. Arthrodeses in functional position of unstable proximal and distal interphalangeal finger joints.

But greater importance is attached to mobilising interventions. Partial or total joint resections are performed, in particular on the elbow and wrist joint, but also especially in the region of the metatarsals. Through this, the fibular deviation of all the toes – frequently associated with pressure ulceration without healing tendency – can be alleviated and an improvement obtained with respect to symptoms, function and appearance.

An extension of resection is interposition arthroplasty. After removal of the different portions of the joint, homologous or autologous tissue (dura, cutis, fascia, fat) is used to cover the bone stumps to prevent bridging of the bones. Immediate introduction of active postoperative exercise therapy also brings good functional results here.

Reconstructive surgery of the locomotor apparatus is today inconceivable without artificial joint replacement in various locations. Even if optimism is somewhat dampened meanwhile, because of the late results, joint replacement surgery frequently brings considerable improvement in the rheumatic patient depending on the local, but also the general, situation.

A patient who has been bedridden for a long time can be mobilised again by endoprosthetic replacement of ankylosed hip joints (with simultaneous anky- losis of the entire vertebral column, the iliosacral joints and also peripheral joints (Fig. 5).

Because of the unfavourable anatomical relations of the knee joint, but also on account of the technical problems, hinge joints do not always offer the best conditions for total substitution of the knee joint. Occasionally, an equally good functional result can be obtained with a partial substitution, e.g. by a sliding prosthesis, with less risk.

Figure 8 shows Swanson's finger joint substitution – here in a psoriatic arthritis with complete fixation of the three ulnar fingers in the closed fist

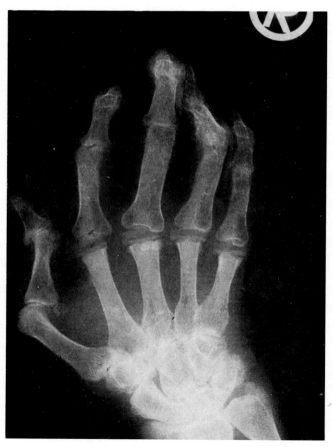

Fig. 8. Swanson replacement of metacarpophalangeal joint II–V.

position and maximal ulnar deviation of the index finger – can achieve an optimal functional result in both hands after 15 years of ankylosis, just like Vainio's interposition arthroplasty. It is done on the other side.

Operative treatment alone is not able to produce an improvement in the condition of the rheumatic patient; it is not a competitor to medicinal and physical therapy, since only an optimal combination of the different therapeutic principles can be successful in the long run.

Antirheumatics are administered at the beginning of the disease for treatment of the symptoms. Cortisone preparations may, when used for stosstherapy, produce a considerable improvement in the condition (Table 1). The medication is maintained preoperatively, then raised to reduce the postoperative oedema.

The inflammation-inhibiting and analgesic effects of corticosteroids often

TABLE 1

Example of short-term oral cortisone stosstherapy (in mg prednisone or prednisolone equivalent doses) with 'steal out' doses

Day	Daily dose (mg)	Reduction (mg)
1–2	25	–
3–4	20	5
5–6	15	5
7–8	10	5
9–10	5	5
11	end of stoss therapy	

lead to the indiscriminate use of these preparations for long term therapy in spite of the considerable side effects. The result is frequently atrophy of the suprarenal glands with defective cortisol formation, so that the patient, as in diabetes mellitus, is dependent on hormonal substitution. It is possible for the damaged suprarenal cortex to recover, but this can only be achieved by a slow reduction of the cortisonoids. This reduction takes place every 3 days by a dose equivalent to 2.5 mg prednisolone until the remaining symptoms appear (Table 2).

To the reduced amount of cortisone is added the highest dose of a non-steroidal symptomatic drug, i.e. about 200 mg indometacin, divided over the day. Then the steroid can be reduced again or totally discontinued. Reduction of the non-steroidal anti-inflammatory agent can take place after the corticoste-

TABLE 2

'Steal out' dosage after long term therapy with high doses of corticosteroids (example: 55–105 days)*: initial dose 30 mg prednisone or prednisolone equivalent dose

Reduction by	Dosage	Duration (days)
5 mg	25 mg/day	5– 7
5 mg	20 mg/day	5– 7
5 mg	15 mg/day	5– 7
2.5 mg	12.5 mg/day	5–14
2.5 mg	10 mg/day	5–14
2.5 mg	7.5 mg/day	5–14
2.5 mg	5 mg/day	5–14
2.5 mg	2.5 mg/day	5–14
2.5 mg every 2nd day	2.5 mg every 2nd day	14

*This Table is not a rigid instruction, but is intended only as a practical guide. Variations are possible to adapt it to the individual reaction of the patient.

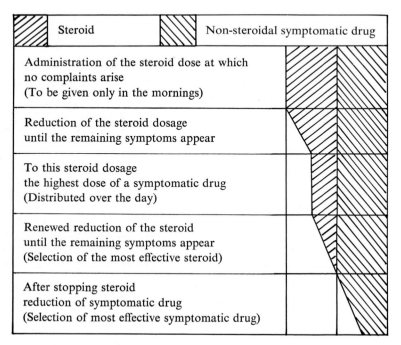

Fig. 9. Steroid reduction plan (Mathies).

roid has been stopped (Fig. 9). The important thing is that the total dose of the corticosteroid is only given in the mornings (= circadian), if possible every second morning (= alternating) even with a double dose. If suprarenal cortical atrophy is present, even if the long term corticosteroid therapy was completed months before, then corticosteroids must be administered before and in stress situations as a vital substitution. Anaesthesia and operations are to be counted as stress situations. The substitution is made preoperatively and intraoperatively by 50–100 mg prednisone-equivalent doses (Fig. 10). Postoperatively, it must be reduced by a half until a dose of 12.5 mg is reached, then the 'steal out' reduc-

Day	Prednisone/Prednisolone Equivalent doses (reduction in brackets)
Last preoperative Operation	1–2 × 25 mg
	1–2 × 50 mg
Postoperative 1– 3	2 × 25 mg daily (– ½) i.v./i.m.
4– 6	25 mg daily (– ½) oral
7– 9	20 mg daily (– 5 mg)
10–12	15 mg daily (– 5 mg)
13–15	12.5 mg daily (– 2.5 mg)
16–18	10 mg daily (– 2.5 mg)
19–21	7.5 mg daily (– 2.5 mg)
22–24	5 mg daily (– 2.5 mg)
25–27	2.5 mg daily (– 2.5 mg)
28th	End of therapy

Fig. 10. Preoperative and postoperative corticosteroid substitution after long term cortisone therapy.

tion of 2.5 mg prednisone-equivalent dose is made every 3 days. Also here, the maintenance or increasing of non-steroidal anti-inflammatory agents is particularly important and spares the use of corticosteroids. Rapid withdrawal of cortisone or deficient intraoperative substitution leads to the cortisone withdrawal syndrome, recognisable by the acute symptoms: rise of temperature, outbreak of sweating, hyperactivity, arthralgias, myalgias and psychic alterations, weakness of concentration, nephelopia, disturbances of accommodation, sensitivity to light, migraine-like headaches, hypotension, syncope, vomiting, diarrhoea, anorexia leading to cachexia and amenorrhoea. The treatment of cortisone withdrawal syndrome is mainly by increased substitution of cortisone (under certain circumstances 100 mg repeated daily several times), and finally by a delayed reduction.

Operative interventions may be able to reduce the inflammatory activity of rheumatoid arthritis. This is expressed also in the possibility of postoperative reduction of the corticosteroids. With reference to the substitution or supplementing of cortisone by indometacin, with its good anti-inflammatory and analgesic effect, we were able to obtain good results, as we have already established in follow-up examinations published a few years ago.

One of our most recent follow-up examinations 7 to 1 year after unilateral and bilateral synovectomy in 58 patients with preoperative high dosage long term cortisone therapy showed that an increase in the cortisone dose was not necessary in a single case (Table 3). In 8 cases it had to be maintained;

TABLE 3

Cortisone administration after synovectomy of the knee joint

Postoperative administration of cortisone	No. of patients after synovectomy of the knee joint		Total no. of patients	%
	Unilateral	Bilateral		
Increased	0	0	0	0
Maintained	4	4	8	13.8
Reduced	5	8	13	22.4
Totally discontinued	24	13	37	63.8
Total	33	25	58	100

in 13 it was reduced. In almost 2/3 of all the patients (37 altogether) it could be stopped altogether. That this reduction of cortisonoids was possible is largely due to the use of operative measures and symptomatic anti-inflammatory and antirheumatic agents together.

Subject index

Prepared by H. Kettner, M.D., Middelburg

hemostasis
complement, 3, 54, 63
inflammation, 45
serotonin, 46
heparin
complement activation, 72
hepatitis
indomethacin side effect,
166
hereditary angioedema
complement, 62
hip osteoarthritis
clinical picture, 130
indomethacin, 156
joint excursion, 132
microtraumatic pain, 157
pain origin, 157
histamine
capillary permeability, 5
complement activation,
62
hyperalgesia, prosta-
glandin, 38
inflammation mediator, 4
pleural exudate, 25
pruritus, prostaglandin
E_1, 38
histamine release
cell cyclic AMP, 5
indomethacin, 17
histology
adjuvant arthritis, 88
Hodgkin disease
fever, indomethacin, 209
hormones
experimental arthritis, 86
horse-radish peroxidase
synovitis, 94
humoral immunity
cell-mediated immunity,
56
5-hydroxytryptamine
see serotonin
hyperalgesia
see also pain and painful
shoulder
bradykinin + prosta-
glandin, 38

histamine + prosta-
glandin, 38
prostaglandin synthesis,
40
prostaglandins, 37
hypertension
bradykinin, 38
prostaglandin, indo-
methacin, 38
prostaglandin release, 38

ibuprofen
rheumatoid arthritis, 201
serum uric acid, 122
immune adherence
complement, 62
phagocytosis, 62
immune complex
complement activation, 57
**immunoglobulin G,
I^{125}-labeled**
vascular permeability, 24
immunoglobulins
complement activation, 57
immunopathology
silicosis adjuvant
arthritis, 90
immunosuppressant agent
carrageenan edema, 36
indomethacin
acetylsalicylic acid,
interaction, 198
ankylosing spondylitis,
156, 185
carrageenan edema, 42
chronic glomerulone-
phritis, 48
chronopharmacology, 99
complement, hemolysis,
71
drug resistance, 170
erythrocyte sedimentation
rate, 198
etiocholanone fever, 217
fibrin adjuvant arthritis,
89
free plasma concentration,
35

gout, 156
histamine release, 17
inflammation model, 16
leukemic fever, 209
long-term therapy, 202
lumbar disc syndrome,
179, 228
osteoarthritis, 156
pharmacokinetics, 165
pharmacological
properties, 225
plasma protein binding,
122
prostaglandin,
hypertension, 38
prostaglandin release,
37, 39, 42
prostaglandin synthetase,
34, 35, 162
rheumatoid arthritis,
167, 175, 197
serum uric acid, 122
soft tissue lesion, 225
temperature regulation,
217
**indomethacin, compared
with:**
acetylsalicylic acid, 198
diazepam, 202
feprazone, 200
ketoprofen, 201
naproxen, 200
oxyphenbutazone, 228
phenylbutazone, 199
sodium salicylate, 199
indomethacin at night
chronopharmacology,
100
morning stiffness, 101
indomethacin plasma level
see plasma indomethacin
indomethacin + prednisone
rheumatoid arthritis, 170
indomethacin side effect
child, 159
diarrhea, 165
dose influence, 189
gastric ulcer, 164